Healthy Aging

Editor

SUSAN M. FRIEDMAN

CLINICS IN GERIATRIC MEDICINE

www.geriatric.theclinics.com

November 2020 • Volume 36 • Number 4

ELSEVIER

1600 John F. Kennedy Boulevard • Suite 1800 • Philadelphia, Pennsylvania, 19103-2899

http://www.theclinics.com

CLINICS IN GERIATRIC MEDICINE Volume 36, Number 4
November 2020 ISSN 0749–0690, ISBN-13: 978-0-323-75720-1

Editor: Katerina Heidhausen
Developmental Editor: Laura Fisher

Clinics in Geriatric Medicine (ISSN 0749-0690) is published quarterly by Elsevier Inc., 360 Park Avenue South, New York, NY 10010-1710. Months of issue are February, May, August, and November. Business and Editorial Offices: 1600 John F. Kennedy Blvd., Suite 1800, Philadelphia, PA 191023-2899. Periodicals postage paid at New York, NY, and additional mailing offices. Subscription prices are $289.00 per year (US individuals), $664.00 per year (US institutions), $100.00 per year (US & Canadian student/resident), $320.00 per year (Canadian individuals), $841.00 per year (Canadian institutions), $414.00 per year (international individuals), $841.00 per year (international institutions), and $195.00 per year (international student/resident). Foreign air speed delivery is included in all Clinics subscription prices. All prices are subject to change without notice. POSTMASTER: Send address changes to Clinics in Geriatric Medicine, Elsevier Health Sciences Division, Subscription Customer Service, 3251 Riverport Lane, Maryland Heights, MO 63043. **Telephone: 1-800-654-2452 (U.S. and Canada); 314-447-8871 (outside U.S. and Canada). Fax: 314-447-8029. E-mail:** journalscustomerservice-usa@elsevier.com **(for print support) or** journalsonlinesupport-usa@elsevier.com **(for online support)**.

Reprints. For copies of 100 or more, of articles in this publication, please contact the Commercial Reprints Department, Elsevier Inc., 360 Park Avenue South, New York, New York 10010-1710. Tel.: 212-633-3874; Fax: 212-633-3820, E-mail: reprints@elsevier.com.

Clinics in Geriatric Medicine is covered in MEDLINE/PubMed (Index Medicus), EMBASE/Excerpta Medica, Current Contents/Clinical Medicine (CC/CM), and the Cumulative Index to Nursing & Allied Health Literature.

Contributors

EDITOR

SUSAN M. FRIEDMAN, MD, MPH, AGSF
Professor of Medicine, University of Rochester School of Medicine and Dentistry, Medical Director, Rochester Lifestyle Medicine Group, Director of Clinical Research, Rochester Lifestyle Medicine Institute, Rochester, New York

AUTHORS

MAYA ABDALLAH, MD
Hematology/Oncology Fellow, Sections of Geriatrics and Hematology/Oncology, Boston University School of Medicine, Boston, Massachusetts

ALI AHMAD, MD
Fellow, Geriatric Medicine, Mayo Clinic College of Medicine and Science, Rochester, Minnesota

LOUISE ARONSON, MD, MFA
Professor of Medicine, Division of Geriatrics, University of California, San Francisco, San Francisco, California

JOHN A. BATSIS, MD, FACP, AGSF, FTOS, FGSA
Section of Weight and Wellness, Department of Medicine, Dartmouth-Hitchcock, Section of General Internal Medicine, Dartmouth-Hitchcock Medical Center, The Dartmouth Institute for Health Policy & Clinical Practice, Lebanon, New Hampshire; Geisel School of Medicine at Dartmouth Hanover, Dartmouth Centers for Health and Aging, Dartmouth College, Hanover, New Hampshire

MARISSA BLACK, MD, MPH
Physician, EvergreenHealth Geriatric Care, Internal Medicine and Geriatrics, Kirkland, Washington; Division of Gerontology and Geriatric Medicine, Clinical Instructor, Department of Medicine, University of Washington, Seattle, Washington

MEGAN BOWMAN, MS, RDN
Clinical Registered Dietitian Nutritionist, Assistant Chief of Nutrition and Food Services, Salt Lake City Veteran Affairs Health Care System, Adjunct Faculty, Department of Exercise Science, Salt Lake Community College, Salt Lake City, Utah

CHRISTINE CIGOLLE, MD
Associate Professor, Division of Geriatric and Palliative Medicine, University of Michigan Medical School, Research Associate Professor, GRECC Ann Arbor Veterans Affairs Hospital, Ann Arbor, Michigan

MARYJO L. CLEVELAND, MD
Associate Professor, Department of Geriatrics and Gerontology, Director, Healthy Aging and Brain Wellness Program, Wake Forest Baptist Health, Sticht Center, Winston-Salem, North Carolina

KATHRYN M. DANIEL, PhD, RN, AGPCNP-BC, GS-C, AGSF, FAAN
Associate Professor, College of Nursing and Health Innovation, The University of Texas at Arlington, Arlington, Texas

ELIZABETH ECKSTROM, MD, MPH
Chief of Geriatrics, Division of General Internal Medicine and Geriatrics, Department of Medicine, Oregon Health & Science University, Portland, Oregon

KATARINA FRIBERG FELSTED, PhD
Associate Professor, Gerontology Interdisciplinary Program, College of Nursing, University of Utah, Salt Lake City, Utah

SUSAN M. FRIEDMAN, MD, MPH, AGSF
Professor of Medicine, University of Rochester School of Medicine and Dentistry, Medical Director, Rochester Lifestyle Medicine Group, Director of Clinical Research, Rochester Lifestyle Medicine Institute, Rochester, New York

SINDHUJA KADAMBI, MD
Fellow, Department of Hematology/Oncology, University of Rochester, Rochester, New York

LEAH KALIN, MD
Assistant Professor, Division of General Internal Medicine and Geriatrics, Department of Medicine, Oregon Health & Science University, Portland, Oregon

HALINA KUSZ, MD, FACP, AGSF
Professor, Department of Medicine, Director of Geriatric Education, Internal Medicine Residency Program, College of Human Medicine, Michigan State University, McLaren Flint, Flint, Michigan

LIANA LIANOV, MD, MPH
Chair, Happiness Science and Positive Health Committee, American College of Lifestyle Medicine, President, Positive Health and Wellness Division, International Positive Psychology Association, Vice-Chair, American Board of Lifestyle Medicine

KAH POH LOH, MBBCh
Senior Instructor, Department of Hematology/Oncology, University of Rochester, Rochester, New York

PAUL MULHAUSEN, MD, FACP, AGSF
Chief Medical Director, Iowa Total Care, Iowa City, Iowa

JENNIFER D. MUNIAK, MD
Assistant Professor of Medicine, Division of Geriatrics, University of Rochester School of Medicine and Dentistry, Rochester, New York

SUVI NEUKAM, DO
Geriatric Fellow, Division of General Internal Medicine and Geriatrics, Department of Medicine, Oregon Health & Science University, Portland, Oregon

VERONICA C. NWAGWU, MD
CWSP, Clinical Assistant Professor, Division of Geriatric and Palliative Medicine, University of Michigan Medical School, Ann Arbor, Michigan

SADHANA PURI, BS
Geisel School of Medicine at Dartmouth Hanover, Hanover, New Hampshire

MEREDITH N. RODERKA, BS
Section of Weight and Wellness, Department of Medicine, Dartmouth-Hitchcock, Lebanon, New Hampshire

NEEMA SHARDA, MD
Assistant Professor, Geriatrics Division, Duke University, Duke University Medical Center, Durham, North Carolina

THEODORE SUH, MD, PhD
Professor of Internal Medicine, Division of Geriatric and Palliative Medicine, University of Michigan Medical School, Professor, GRECC Ann Arbor Veterans Affairs Hospital, Ann Arbor, Michigan

HEIDI WHITE, MD, MHS, MEd
Professor, Geriatrics Division, Duke University, Duke University Medical Center, Durham, North Carolina

SERENA WONG, DO
Medical Instructor, Geriatrics Division, Duke University, Duke University Medical Center, Durham, North Carolina

JESSICA WRIGHT, PA-C
Clinical Instructor, Division of General Internal Medicine and Geriatrics, Department of Medicine, Oregon Health & Science University, Portland, Oregon

Contents

Preface: Healthy Aging: What Do We Mean, and How Do We Accomplish It? xiii

Susan M. Friedman

Healthy Aging Across the Stages of Old Age 549

Louise Aronson

Healthy aging is among the key frontiers for twenty-first century geriatrics and gerontology. Gerontology is positioned to address not only disease, debility, frailty, and death but also patients' hopes to remain healthy and high functioning and optimize their wellness. Definitions, models, and metrics of healthy aging are increasingly dynamic and multidimensional, drawing from biomedicine, social sciences, older adults' perspectives, and geroscience. Given current and projected demographics, focus on healthy aging at population, health system, research, clinical, and individual levels will lower costs and burdens while improving lives. Multiple models and strategies exist to guide progress in this critical emerging area.

How Do Geriatric Principles Inform Healthy Aging? 559

Jennifer D. Muniak and Paul Mulhausen

Healthy aging long has been held as a core belief and priority of geriatrics, yet clinical, scholarly, and advocacy efforts have not kept pace with attention to multimorbidity and end-of-life care. With an aging US population and trends toward higher rates of lifestyle diseases, there is imperative for geriatricians to engage in efforts to promote healthy aging. Lifestyle medicine offers an evidence-based approach to healthy aging at any point in the life span. This emerging branch of medical practice has synergistic principles and frameworks with the field of geriatrics, which should further empower geriatricians to engage in promoting healthy aging.

Multimorbidity, Function, and Cognition in Aging 569

Sindhuja Kadambi, Maya Abdallah, and Kah Poh Loh

Multimorbidity is a global health challenge. Here, we define multimorbidity, describe ways multimorbidity is measured, discuss the prevalence of multimorbidity and how it differs across different populations, examine mechanisms of disease and disability, and discuss the effects of multimorbidity on outcomes such as survival and function.

Preserving Cognition, Preventing Dementia 585

Maryjo L. Cleveland

Dementia incidence continues to rise in the United States and around the world. Although age is the single biggest risk factor for the development of dementia, it is not considered normal sequelae of aging. Although there has been little to no progress made in the past couple of decades in the treatment or cure of Alzheimer disease, there has been significant progress made in prevention. Single factors, such as hearing loss or cardiovascular risk factors, may increase the risk for cognitive decline. The opportunity to mitigate these risk factors provides an exciting new healthy aging approach to dementia prevention.

Preserving Engagement, Nurturing Resilience   601

Halina Kusz and Ali Ahmad

Engagement and resilience constitute 2 psychological aspects of healthy aging that are commonly identified by many individuals as more important than health or longevity. Both of them play a crucial role in healthy aging. Social engagement enhances psychological well-being and improves physical and cognitive health outcomes. In times of adversity, resilience buffers the negative effects of stress and promotes return to baseline health and function. Strong resilience helps individuals become more engaged and active engagement promotes resilience. We discuss the role, health outcomes, and practical implications of these 2 major domains of healthy aging.

Reducing Frailty to Promote Healthy Aging   613

Veronica C. Nwagwu, Christine Cigolle, and Theodore Suh

Frailty is a complex geriatric syndrome. Frail patients typically present with an array of multiple complex symptoms and significantly reduced tolerance for medical and surgical interventions. A multidomain approach is required to effectively treat/manage frailty.

Addressing Obesity to Promote Healthy Aging   631

Meredith N. Roderka, Sadhana Puri, and John A. Batsis

The population worldwide is aging and prevalence of obesity in this population is increasing. The range of consequences that effect these at-risk patients include increased risk of falls, fractures, reduced quality of life, and cognitive decline. This article describes the epidemiology of obesity, risks and benefits of weight loss, and importance of treating obesity to help promote healthy aging. Health care professionals should encourage older adults with obesity to implement healthy lifestyle behaviors including exercise and diet routine. Treating obesity in older adults mitigates the significant public health crisis, and reduces health care utilization and risk of long-term adverse events.

Lifestyle (Medicine) and Healthy Aging   645

Susan M. Friedman

Healthy aging is a process that occurs over the life cycle. Health habits established early and practiced throughout life impact longevity, the ability to reach old age, and the health with which one experiences older adulthood. The new field of lifestyle medicine addresses root causes of disease by targeting nutrition, physical activity, well-being, stress management, substance use, connectedness, and sleep. As a result, lifestyle medicine can optimize the trajectory of aging, and promote targets that have been recognized in geriatric medicine as essential to well-being and quality of life, resulting in a compression of morbidity.

Nutrition and Healthy Aging   655

Marissa Black and Megan Bowman

Diet is a key determinant of health and is vital to the prevention and management of chronic disease. The predictors of an individual's dietary health are complex and influenced by multiple socioeconomic, environmental, and behavioral domains. Dietary behavior change in late life requires an in-depth understanding of internal and external factors influencing the individual and knowledge of community resources available. Dietary patterns—the combination of foods and beverages consumed—may be related to quality of life and health in older adults. Dietary patterns may also be easier for individuals to adopt and understand than dietary planning based on single nutrients.

Physical Activity and Healthy Aging   671

Elizabeth Eckstrom, Suvi Neukam, Leah Kalin, and Jessica Wright

Healthy aging is the ability to maintain independence, purpose, vitality, and quality of life into old age despite unexpected medical conditions, accidents, and unhelpful social determinants of health. Exercise, or physical activity, is an important component of healthy aging, preventing or mitigating falls, pain, sarcopenia, osteoporosis, and cognitive impairment. A well-balanced exercise program includes daily aerobic, strength, balance, and flexibility components. Most older adults do not meet the currently recommended minutes of regular physical activity weekly. Counseling by health care providers may help older adults improve exercise habits, but it is also important to take advantage of community-based exercise opportunities.

Mindfulness, Stress, and Aging   685

Katarina Friberg Felsted

Mindfulness has been applied in several adaptations, including Mindfulness-Based Stress Reduction and Mindfulness-Based Cognitive Therapy, to treat chronic conditions in older adults. Older adults may be particularly well suited for mindfulness interventions, because they bring decades of life experience to this contemplative therapy. Mindfulness is also an appealing intervention for older adults as it is inexpensive, effective over time, and easy to access. This article examines mental and physical chronic conditions proven responsive to mindfulness, including cognitive function, anxiety, depression, sleep quality, loneliness, posttraumatic stress disorder, cardiovascular conditions, diabetes, rheumatoid arthritis, Parkinson's disease, urge urinary incontinence, and chronic pain.

The Role of Prevention in Healthy Aging   697

Neema Sharda, Serena Wong, and Heidi White

This article explores the role of prevention in healthy aging from the perspective of individualized prevention in the clinic and population-based prevention with system-level support. The traditional medical model has significant limitations to effectively target impactful outcomes related to geriatric syndromes that encompass debility, frequent hospitalizations, loss of independence, and disease progression. This article reviews aspects of the clinic visit and subsequent interventions, such as immunizations and screenings, that promote disease and disability prevention. Finally, we review the value of Population Health Management as a model of care for delivering population-based, system-level supported, patient-centered health care plans.

Best Practices for Promoting Healthy Aging   713

Kathryn M. Daniel

This article outlines key well-known population health practices at the community level that benefit all members of the community, especially older adults.

Getting from Here to There: Motivational Interviewing and Other Techniques to Promote Healthy Aging   719

Liana Lianov

Successful health behavior change relies on the autonomy of the individual who is driven toward personally meaningful, positive goals. The medical practitioner and health care team can use several techniques to facilitate such change effectively, including motivational interviewing, cognitive behavioral restructuring, appreciative inquiry, and positive psychology techniques. Older adults can be supported to make change, and may have greater capacity to maintain those changes due to increased levels of conscientiousness. Positive psychology approaches may be effective in older adults, due to evidence that, as individuals age, they tend to prioritize activities that bring them satisfaction and emotional well-being.

CLINICS IN GERIATRIC MEDICINE

FORTHCOMING ISSUES

February 2021
Gastroenterology
Amir E. Soumekh and Philip O. Katz, *Editors*

May 2021
Sleep in the Elderly
Steven H. Feinsilver and Margarita Oks, *Editors*

August 2021
Peripheral Nerve Disease in the Geriatric Population
Peter Jin, *Editor*

RECENT ISSUES

August 2020
Diabetes in Older Adults
S. Sethu K. Reddy, *Editor*

May 2020
Geriatric Psychiatry
Dan G. Blazer and Susan K. Schultz, *Editors*

February 2020
Parkinson Disease
Carlos Singer and Stephen Reich, *Editors*

SERIES OF RELATED INTEREST

Medical Clinics of North America
Primary Care: Clinics in Office Practice

THE CLINICS ARE AVAILABLE ONLINE!
Access your subscription at:
www.theclinics.com

Preface

Healthy Aging: What Do We Mean, and How Do We Accomplish It?

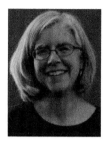

Susan M. Friedman, MD, MPH, AGSF
Editor

"It's not the years in your life that count. It's the life in your years." This quote, or a variant of it, has been attributed to Adlai Stevenson, Abraham Lincoln, Dr Edward Stieglitz, and others. It is a goal that is central to Geriatric Medicine: the idea of maintaining vitality throughout the life course. But healthy aging is a complex construct, which differs between individuals and between populations and cultures, and also changes over time within an individual. It incorporates concepts that are more traditional to Medicine, such as preventing and treating illness; ideas that are important in Geriatrics, like preserving function, cognition, and quality of life; and values that resonate with older adults, like maintaining a sense of purpose, having meaningful relationships, and being able to live according to one's values.

We know that the aging experience can be impacted significantly by a person's life course, which includes lifestyle. Science is showing the power of healthy lifestyle to increase longevity, compress morbidity, and facilitate a broad definition of health, that encompasses not only avoiding or delaying disease but also living a life of meaning, joy, dignity, gratitude, and connectedness.

In this issue on healthy aging, we bring together concepts from 2 disciplines: the tenet of Geriatrics that works with patients at whatever point they are in their lives, to understand and then foster their goals, and the focus of Lifestyle Medicine, which seeks to develop systems and interventions that help to reduce the impact of chronic disease, by delaying onset, reducing severity, and even reversing chronic illness. It is my hope that the efforts of these 2 fields, which each push the boundaries of current health care, can connect in a way that improves the opportunities for all to live a healthy life.

Two elegant conceptual articles start this discussion. Dr Aronson writes about untangling concepts like usual versus normal aging, and healthy versus successful aging; and how the goals of healthy aging change across the stages of old age, and when

Clin Geriatr Med 36 (2020) xiii–xiv
https://doi.org/10.1016/j.cger.2020.08.001
0749-0690/20/© 2020 Published by Elsevier Inc.

viewed from a population level down to the level of the individual. Drs Muniak and Mulhausen articulate the principles of Geriatrics that can be applied to healthy aging and addressing lifestyle, such as an appreciation of and comfort with complexity and holistic thinking, a focus on personal interactions, an understanding of the patient's biopsychosocial circumstances, and a focus on goals and motivation.

We then turn to a discussion of the components outlined in the Rowe and Kahn model of successful aging, as Dr Kadambi and colleagues discuss the interaction of multimorbidity, functional decline, and cognition; Dr Cleveland presents evidence on preventing dementia, and Drs Kusz and Ahmad review issues of preserving engagement and nurturing resilience. Dr Nwagwu and colleagues address an issue central to Geriatrics, namely, frailty, and Ms Roderka and colleagues present an issue that is increasingly impacting the aging experience: obesity.

The next section discusses Lifestyle Medicine and reviews evidence of how it impacts healthy aging. Several of the pillars of Lifestyle Medicine are then addressed: Dr Black and Ms Bowman discuss nutrition; Dr Eckstrom and colleagues discuss physical activity, and Dr Friberg Felsted addresses mindfulness and stress. The next 2 articles discuss the need to broaden our approach to promoting wellness through our focus on systems: Dr Sharda and colleagues address an expanded approach to prevention beyond a primarily medical model, and Dr Daniel discusses best practices that promote healthy aging. Finally, Dr Lianov presents an overview of how to work with patients to help them make and sustain changes that will foster healthy aging.

The current medical system does not optimally promote healthy aging, but we have an opportunity to change this by developing health-enhancing networks that foster this outcome. Healthy aging can best be achieved by an integration of efforts: from the population, to the health care system, to the individual. We need a change in medical culture and resource allocation in order to do this. The fields of Geriatric and Lifestyle Medicine, which each have a history of embracing system change to improve outcomes for our patients, can develop synergistic efforts to promote healthy aging for all. The time is now!

Susan M. Friedman, MD, MPH, AGSF
University of Rochester School
of Medicine and Dentistry
Rochester Lifestyle Medicine
Highland Hospital
1000 South Avenue, Box 58
Rochester, NY 14620, USA

E-mail address:
Susan_Friedman@urmc.rochester.edu

Healthy Aging Across the Stages of Old Age

Louise Aronson, MD, MFA

KEYWORDS

- Healthy aging • Health promotion • Prevention • Health span • Longevity
- Successful aging

KEY POINTS

- There is no consensus definition of healthy aging, but the most useful definitions are dynamic and multifactorial, including physical, social, mental and spiritual wellness, function, adaptation, social connectedness, and meaning.
- Although the terms healthy aging and successful aging have been used interchangeably, they can and should be distinguished in research and clinical care.
- Population-level goals of healthy aging must include health system transformation, age-friendly environments, comprehensive long-term care, and universal standards.
- Individual-level goals of healthy aging move beyond disease and symptom management to lifelong cognitive, physical, mental, and social health promotion and reprioritization of social policies and clinical encounters.
- Expanding geriatrics to include healthy aging with help the field to serve all older adults, recruit more health professionals, and fulfill its core mission.

Healthy aging has been seen as a goal, physiologic state, psychological approach, marketing tool, and scientific frontier. For some, the term constitutes an oxymoron. After all, the word *healthy* usually implies optimal function and freedom from disease, whereas *aging* is associated with illness and the loss of vitality and abilities. In geriatrics and related disciplines, the phrase *healthy aging* increasingly signals opportunities to positively and proactively impact wellness throughout old age. Although life expectancy nearly doubled in the twentieth century, the ratio of health span (healthy years of life) to life span (total years alive) decreased. Old age became associated with multimorbidity, functional decline, and dependency, and the field of geriatrics prioritized the care of the oldest, sickest, and frailest old patients. That approach was both pragmatic and in keeping with a laudable mission of social justice for the most vulnerable older adults. More recently, however, the field's narrow lens has been seen as

Division of Geriatrics, University of California, San Francisco, 3333 California Street, Suite 380, San Francisco, CA 94143, USA
E-mail address: Louise.aronson@ucsf.edu
Twitter: @louisearonson (L.A.)

Clin Geriatr Med 36 (2020) 549–558
https://doi.org/10.1016/j.cger.2020.06.001
0749-0690/20/© 2020 The Author. Published by Elsevier Inc. All rights reserved.

misaligned with our core mission to provide care across the decades and substages of old age.[1]

In the twenty-first century, people of all ages, including older adults, routinely feel and seem to be healthy despite having 1 or many chronic diseases.[2] As a result, more health professionals are taking a broader view of health, one that moves beyond the 1948 World Health Organization definition of health as "a state of complete physical, mental and social well-being and not merely the absence of disease or infirmity."[3] For some, the term *wellness* better captures that broader approach, but others believe the word *health* can and should allow for a sense of "physical, mental and social well-being" despite what some might perceive as serious illness or debilities. In either case, by focusing more on healthy aging within geriatrics, we will be better positioned to incorporate cutting-edge geroscience into clinical care; attend to prevention, health promotion, and wellness not just disease and frailty; appeal to trainees with wider ranges of interests; and, most important, more fully respond to the needs and goals of all older patients as they move through the decades of old age. As the 2018 American Geriatrics Society White Paper on Healthy Aging stated: "Promotion of a realistic, dynamic, multidimensional view of healthy aging is an important goal obtainable through traditional and innovative models of health promotion and prevention."[4]

DEFINITIONS

What constitutes healthy aging varies with time period and vantage point. The media portrays healthy aging as akin to pornography: people know it when they see it. According to this definition, a healthy ager is an older person who moves and thinks quickly and easily, who "looks young," and who is actively engaged across many sectors of life: work, exercise, family, and community.[5] Such people defy stereotypes, living an old age that almost everyone hopes for and few people attain. Among the key arguments for widespread incorporation of healthy aging into health care and geriatrics health professions is to dramatically increase the number of people across socioeconomic, racial, gender, religious, ethnic, age, and ability lines with opportunities for healthy aging.

In the medical literature, healthy aging has sometimes been used interchangeably with successful aging, a decades-old concept discussed in greater detail in the next section. Other descriptors include optimal, positive, productive, effective, and active. Biomedical scientists and clinicians have traditionally considered successful aging as the absence of disease and physical or cognitive disabilities. Social scientists tend to see it as an old age of well-being, socialization, and life satisfaction and emphasize the need to include older adults' own criteria. Other scholars note the importance of making the maintenance of positive health not merely the avoidance of pathology as the defining trait, as well as incorporating both objective and subjective dimensions into the definition.[6,7]

Older adults' definitions of healthy aging are closer to those of social and behavioral scientists than health professionals. For them, healthy aging is not a singular outcome or the absence of changes compared with younger years. Instead, healthy means having adapted to aging in ways that the person finds acceptable and includes personal, familial and spiritual domains.[8] This definition is analogous to the biomedical literature's usage of "well-being" and is distinctly person centered, because "acceptable" will vary according to the person's psyche and sociocultural circumstances, not just their traditional health metrics. In 1 community-based study, older adults defined health as the ability to go and do something meaningful.[9] Accomplishing that did not preclude disease or debility, but did have 4 sociopersonal requirements: having something worthwhile to do, the abilities to overcome challenges, the necessary external resources to support the activity, and the will to go and do it. In this view, health did not enable the meaningful activity; rather, it resulted from it.

Although focused on successful not healthy aging, a study that included both Japanese-American and white American cohorts from King County, Washington, noted that older adults defined successful aging as a broader, more multidimensional process than researchers did, incorporating physical, psychological, social, and functional health.[10] Similarly, a California-based study of Korean, Vietnamese, and Latino elders found that, despite different cultures, each believed healthy aging required not only good physical and mental health, but also optimism and acceptance of changes, social connectedness, taking charge of one's health, and independence and self-worth.[11] In general, older adults put greater value on social engagement and personal resources, such as attitude as markers of success with aging, than the physical function or longevity measures often prioritized in research studies of the topic.[12]

In recent years, leading health organizations have adopted definitions of healthy aging that incorporate key attributes of the biomedical, social science, and older adult definitions. Health Canada describes healthy aging as, "a lifelong process of optimizing opportunities for improving and preserving health and physical, social and mental wellness, independence, quality of life and enhancing successful life-course transitions."[13] The World Health Organization defines healthy aging as, "the process of developing and maintaining the functional ability that enables well-being in old age."[14] They additionally note that functional ability depends on both intrinsic and environmental characteristics and that it is present when a person is able to be and do what they value. Being free of disease and debility are not requirements and the goal is to optimize "opportunities for health, participation and security in order to enhance quality of life as people age."[15]

In summary, definitions of healthy aging are varied and include high physical, cognitive, and social functioning; adaptation to age-related changes; the avoidance of morbidity and disability; and self-perception of health or well-being. As of early 2020, no consensus definition of healthy aging exists.

MODELS OF HEALTHY AGING

Healthy aging has been a concern of human societies for millennia. Methods for longer, healthier lives were mentioned in the ancient medical writings of China, Egypt, Greece, Rome, and what is now Iran. More recently, an array of conceptual frameworks of healthy aging have emerged with emphases that range from the biomedical to the psychosocial and multidimensional (**Table 1**).[16]

Biomedical Model

Perhaps the most well-known healthy aging model was first advanced in 1987 when geriatrician John W. Rowe and social psychologist Robert L. Kahn published a paradigm-shifting paper in *Science* entitled, "Healthy Aging: Usual and Successful." Based on their work with the longitudinal MacArthur Foundation Study on Successful Aging, Rowe and Kahn argued that the methods and assumptions of aging researchers across disciplines had led to the erroneous conclusion that usual aging, with its inexorable accumulation of debilities and diseases, was natural and immutable. "Normal aging" actually included actually included 2 very different groups: large numbers of people undergoing usual aging and smaller numbers who might be said to be successfully aging.

Table 1			
Examples of leading models of successful aging			
Approach	**Authors**	**Key Components**	**Definition of Success**
Biomedical	Rowe & Kahn,[17] 1997	1. Being free of disease and disability 2. Having high cognitive and physical abilities 3. Interacting with others in meaningful ways	All 3 are present
Psychosocial	Baltes & Baltes,[21] 1990	• Selection of desirable, feasible goals • Optimization: engaging in behaviors that maximize available resources, internal and external • Compensation: choosing alternative means of reaching goal despite limitations	Using these 3 processes to maximize gains and minimize losses over time
Multidimensional	Young et al,[27] 2009	• Physiologic: disease and function • Psychological: coping, emotional vitality, resilience • Sociologic: engagement with life and spirituality	Scored on a 0–5 scale, from less to more success in 5 variables: disease, function, cognition, vitality, and engagement

For decades, studies of human aging had compared physiologic and psychological variables among age groups to separate the impact of disease from that of so-called normal aging. The inadvertent consequence of this approach was relative inattention to the considerable heterogeneity of those same variables among the individuals within each aging cohort, a choice that led to the conflation of the way most people aged with the aging process itself. Because of this methodologic artifact, clinicians, academics, and the general public believed that intrinsic factors such as genetics were the primary determinant of the deficits and losses commonly seen in older adults. The critical role of extrinsic factors such as diet, physical activity, habits, and attitudes on late life development was overlooked. By examining nondiseased cohorts for those older adults with minimal losses, the successful agers, the MacArthur Foundation study revealed the significant personal, behavioral, and psychosocial contributors to the aging process. Usual aging, it seemed, could be modified by lifestyle and state of mind to decrease older people's risk of disease and debility. Changes once considered age intrinsic were in fact age related and modifiable.

Rowe and Kahn's model of successful aging has 3 main attributes: (1) being free of disease and disability, (2) having high cognitive and physical abilities, and (3) interacting with others in meaningful ways. In subsequent work, they elaborated the contributors and components of each but the model, although still widely referenced, also continues to generate controversy.[17] It has been criticized for its overemphasis on individual control and its inadequate accounting for structural and cultural determinants of health, aging biology, spirituality, and subjective criteria of success.[18–20] Additionally, it is considered static, the assessment of successful versus usual aging measured at a given moment in time, whereas aging itself is dynamic and developmental.

Psychosocial Model

The psychology literature takes a life course approach to models of healthy aging. Viewing aging as a lifelong process, models in this tradition allow for continuity and change across the lifespan and growth and adaptation at all ages. They move beyond the Rowe and Kahn emphasis on personal agency to consider the impact of historical, social, and cultural forces on individual aging. The most well-known such model is Baltes and Baltes' selection–optimization–compensation (SOC). It posits the presence of 3 interacting elements—selection, optimization, and compensation—that allow individuals to age successfully throughout the lifespan, adjusting their goals and aspirations to ensure ongoing fit with their physiologic and functional status.[21] Where Rowe and Kahn's model articulated what they believed successful aging looked like, Baltes and Baltes emphasized how a person might age successfully, providing dynamic strategies for life management that might lead to satisfaction across contexts and the substages of old age.

In the SOC model, *selection* involves deciding on goals in ways that are either elective or desirable yet feasible path in the context of their available internal and external resources, which may include physical, functional, sociocultural, and economic restrictions. *Optimization* occurs when the person engages in behaviors that augment those available resources and maximize their ability to successfully meet their chosen goals. Finally, *compensation* takes place when the person actively chooses alternative means of achieving their goals when their losses and limitations mean they can no longer achieve the goal by previous means. Subsequent studies have provided evidence that the SOC model correlates with successful development across the life span. For people already in old age, Freund and Baltes provided evidence for associations between the SOC components and various indicators of subjective well-being, including positive emotions, autonomy, environmental mastery, personal growth, positive relations, purpose in life, and self-acceptance.[22]

Other scholars outside biomedicine have proposed theories of successful aging that do not require the absence of disease or debility but healthy adaptation to it. These include Carstensen's socioemotional selectivity theory, which says older adults create positive experiences by prioritizing emotional goals and adjusting social interactions to help meet them.[23] Kahana and Kahana's stress theory based model similarly posits success as achieving quality of life despite illness and social and functional losses.[24] By drawing on internal psychoemotional and external social resources, they suggest that older adults can adapt, improve their own health, recruit support, and plan future adaptations so as to retain agency and meet goals. These adaptation-based models of healthy aging notwithstanding, a 2009 review of data-based successful aging studies noted that most used definitions primarily based on the absence of disability with only a minority also including either psychosocial variables or positive phenomena, such as attitude or adaptation.[25] A second review further highlighted the gulf between researcher and lay definitions.[26] Moreover, depending on how successful aging was defined and which measurements were used, its prevalence ranged from 0.4% to 95% across the 28 studies included in the analysis.

Multidimensional Models

In response to this diversity of models and metrics, Young and colleagues[27,28] developed and validated a novel multidimensional construct of successful aging that allowed for the coexistence of "success" and chronic disease. They argue that because aging is heterogeneous, there can be no single definition of or pathway to success. This model has 3 domains: (1) physiologic—the absence of diseases and functional impairments, (2) psychological—cognitive function, emotional vitality, coping, resilience, and (3) social—engagement with life, spirituality, and the use of social support mechanisms for adaptation. A person can be successful in any 1 or 2 domains, with the most successful achieving highest scores in all 3. Unlike most others, Young and colleagues' model allows for varied degrees and types of success; it accommodates both physically healthy people with psychological or social challenges and people with age-related limitations as long as they are able to invoke psychological and social compensation, as well as people with partial limitations in each domain. Successful aging occurs whenever a person has high well-being, quality of life, and personal fulfilment.

DILEMMAS, SOLUTIONS, AND OPPORTUNITIES

Definitions and models of healthy aging are only useful insofar as they inform clinical care, professional education, medical research and human lives. At present, the 2 highest frequency terms are "successful aging" and "healthy aging," and they are often used interchangeably. The American Geriatrics Society Healthy Aging White Paper raised the related question of whether the term healthy aging should be inclusive, with the ability to encompass well-being among older adults of all ages and functional abilities, or exclusive and used to enact social, health care, and lifestyle changes that promote optimal health.[4] McLaughlin and colleagues[29] offered a solution, arguing that a distinction can be made between successful and healthy aging, with successful aging requiring the absence of disease, whereas healthy aging does not. In essence, healthy aging becomes the inclusive term, a goal present across the substages of old age, whereas successful aging signals optimal human health and functioning. This approach, although imperfect, encompasses the existing literature while allowing progress in the study and care of both optimal agers and all older adults at all ages and physiologic, psychological, and social functional levels. Although the word success cannot be applied to aging without also invoking failure—a risky endeavor given the world's uneven playing fields and the inevitability of physiologic decline and death—it will be hard to remove it from either the literature or the popular lexicon after decades of use.

Notably, none of the most widely used models of healthy aging incorporate objective markers of aging. As precision medicine and geroscience become more prominent in clinical care and research, this is likely to change. Molecular biomarkers that might be considered in future models include telomere length, DNA repair, epigenetic modification via DNA methylation, transcriptome profiles, insulin/insulin-like growth factor 1 signaling, mechanistic target of rapamycin protein, advanced glycation end-products, microRNAs, NAD+, and the sirtuins.[30] In geriatrics, we also have established phenotypic markers with proven predictive value that might inform healthy aging interventions. These include gait speed, grip strength, lower extremity function, muscle mass, body mass index, and waist circumference, among many others.[31–33] Preliminary studies suggest such markers may not measure the same aspects of the aging process, so further studies should be done before incorporating these metrics into existing or novel models.[34]

Another challenge to the application of healthy aging models across the substages of old age is that such stages are not only poorly defined, but are not infrequently fluid. An old person undergoing chemotherapy or severe family stress may seem to be older and frailer 1 year and once through those traumas in subsequent years may seem "younger" again. Where childhood and adulthood generally progress in a uniform fashion from infant to teen or young adult to middle age, we lack both that clear trajectory and a language for how people progress through elderhood. Nevertheless, existing frameworks provide guidance for how clinicians can categorize patient health status to inform goal setting. In the 1980s, then Suzman and Riley added the "oldest old" to Neugarten's framework of "young old" and "old-old" based on associations between psychological state and chronologic age.[35,36] Although that approach seems to be out of line with the functional status approach of geriatrics, it has the advantage of easy applicability by professionals and the lay public. Indeed, it might be said to have informed the World Health Organization's identification of 3 subpopulations of older people: those with relatively high and stable capacity, those with decreasing capacity, and those with substantial losses of capacity.[37] Walter and Covinsky's model[38] of cancer screening offers a more medical approach, categorizing individual health based on their life expectancy (informed by disease and functional status), benefits and harms of the intervention, and patient values and preferences. Their work has been incorporated into geriatric practice beyond its initial application, with clinicians assessing diverse risk–benefit ratios with their patients based on life expectancy, multimorbidity, function, and patient goals.

GOALS OF HEALTHY AGING ACROSS THE STAGES OF OLD AGE

Goal setting operationalizes definitions and models. At the population level, the World Health Organization proposes that public health action for healthy aging should focus on building abilities in individuals and their environments so older adults can navigate changing circumstances by innovating novel ways of functioning.[37] They advocate the following goals: (1) align health systems with the older populations they now serve, with less focus on diseases, symptoms, acute care, and cure and more on function and chronic care; (2) develop comprehensive long-term care systems that minimize dependence, free women from career-ending caregiving and families from catastrophic costs, and support older adults' basic rights and dignity; (3) age-friendly environments; and (4) the development of universal metrics and monitoring systems.

At the health system level, the American Geriatrics Society White Paper advocates an approach of primary (preventing risk factors and disease onset), secondary (preventing disease progression), and tertiary (limiting impairments, disabilities and complications) prevention. Although the language here takes the traditional negative medical framing—preventing the bad rather than promoting the good, their 5 specific strategies, based on the National Prevention Council's Healthy Aging Strategy, move the discussion of healthy aging forward into the positive, with only the first reflecting conventional medicine's usual approach[39]: (1) promoting health, preventing injury, and managing chronic conditions, (2) optimizing cognitive health, (3) optimizing physical health, (4) optimizing mental health, and (5) facilitating social engagement.

At the individual level, it will be essential to simultaneously take a patient-centered approach and work to counter sociocultural messaging that usual aging is biologically predetermined and only minimally modifiable by policies, communities, and lifestyle. This task will be particularly paramount for patients from populations where high risk for unhealthy aging begins in utero and extends through childhood as a result of economic and social inequities. To ensure their priorities are met, clinicians should ask all old patients new sets of questions, including: What gives your life meaning? What gives you joy? Describe how you have adapted to a change or loss in the past? Tell me about a time when you did something that made you feel healthier? Who are the important people and groups in your life?

MOVING FORWARD

Healthy aging is among the key frontiers for twenty-first century geriatrics and geron-tology. With a broader definition of geriatric medicine and increased training in strate-gies to promote, maintain and restore health and wellness, the field will be position to address not only disease, debility, frailty, and death but also patients' hopes to remain healthy and high functioning for as long as possible and optimize their wellness there-after. In recent decades, we have been good citizens of the larger health care system that overvalues the treatment of disease, reducing prevention to little more than vacci-nation and cancer screening. In response, both patients and clinicians have looked elsewhere for information and support. The American Academy of Anti-Aging Medi-cine, with its stated focus on the optimization of human aging, claims 4 times as many members as the American Geriatrics Society, and older patients in significant numbers are turning to integrative medicine modalities to meet health promotion and disease management needs not addressed by conventional medical care.[40] Only very recently has healthy aging, in all its diversity, begun to enter the arenas of geriatrics training, practice, and research.

Healthy aging will not be possible without a wholesale rethinking of what we currently call health care, moving beyond medical treatment to comprehensive care for human health. This will require culture change, both within medicine and more generally. People of all ages cannot attain health without opportunities for social engagement, physical activity, agency and personal growth. Although biology plays a role in aging, it is far from the only determinant of a person's chance of healthy aging. Although younger age correlates with health, so too do socioeconomics (early life, ed-ucation, mid-life economic status), behavior (smoking, physical activity, diet, alcohol) and psychosocial situation (stress, social engagement, resilience).[41–43] Human beings need opportunities, meaning, purpose and responsibility across the lifespan, even when the means of achieving them varies by culture, between individuals, and over the lifespan. Given the priorities of aging Baby Boomers and our stated goal as pro-fessionals to improve the lives of older adults, geriatric medicine can and should be a leader in this transformation.

DISCLOSURE

The author has nothing to disclose.

REFERENCES

1. Friedman SM, Shah K, Hall WJ. Failing to focus on healthy aging: a frailty of our discipline? J Am Geriatr Soc 2015;63(7):1459–62.
2. Fallon CK, Karlawish J. Is the WHO definition of health aging well? Frameworks for "Health" after three score and ten. Am J Public Health 2019;109:1104–6.
3. Official Records of WHO, no. 2, p. 100, entered into force on 7 April 1948. Avail-able at: https://www.who.int/governance/eb/who_constitution_en.pdf. Accessed January 26, 2020.
4. Friedman SM, Mulhausen P, Cleveland ML, et al. Healthy aging: American Geri-atrics Society white paper executive summary. J Am Geriatr Soc 2018;67:17–20.
5. Lamb S. Successful aging as a contemporary obsession: global perspectives. New Brunswick (NJ): Rutgers University Press; 2017.
6. Kaplan MS, Huguet N, Orpana H, et al. Prevalence and factors associated with thriving in older adulthood: a 10-year population-based study. J Gerontol A Biol Sci Med Sci 2008;63(10):1097–104.

7. Pruchno RA, Wilson-Genderson M, Rose M, et al. Successful aging: early influences and contemporary characteristics. Gerontologist 2010;50(6):821–33.
8. Hung L, Kempen GIJM, DeVries NK. Cross-cultural comparison between academic and lay views of healthy ageing: a literature review. Ageing Soc 2010;30:1371–91.
9. Bryant LL, Corbett KK, Kutner JS. In their own words: a model of healthy aging. Soc Sci Med 2001;53(7):927–41.
10. Phelan EA, Anderson LA, LaCroix AZ, et al. Older adults' views of "successful aging"—how do they compare with researchers' definitions? J Am Geriatr Soc 2004;52:211–6.
11. Nguyen H, Lee JA, Sorkin DH, et al. "Living happily despite having an illness": perceptions of healthy aging among Korean American, Vietnamese American, and Latino older adults. Appl Nurs Res 2019;48:30–6.
12. Cosco TD, Prina AM, Perales J, et al. Lay perspectives of successful ageing: a systematic review and meta-ethnography. BMJ Open 2013;3(6).
13. Health Canada. Workshop on healthy aging 2001. Available at: http://publications.gc.ca/collections/Collection/H39-612-2002-1E.pdf. Accessed January 26, 2020.
14. What is healthy ageing. Available at: http://www.who.int/ageing/healthy-ageing/en/. Accessed January 4, 2020.
15. World Health Organization. Active ageing: a policy framework 2002. Available at: https://extranet.who.int/agefriendlyworld/wp-content/uploads/2014/06/WHO-Active-Ageing-Framework.pdf. Accessed January 4, 2020.
16. Martin P, Kelly N, Kahana B, et al. Defining successful aging: a tangible or elusive concept? Gerontologist 2015;55:14–25.
17. Rowe JW, Kahn RL. Successful aging. Gerontologist 1997;37:433–41.
18. Stowe JD, Cooney TM. Examining Rowe and Kahn's concept of successful aging: importance of taking a life course perspective. Gerontologist 2015;55(1):43–50.
19. Crowther MR, Parker MW, Achenbaum WA, et al. Rowe and Kahn's model of successful aging revisited: positive spirituality—the forgotten factor. Gerontologist 2002;42(5):613–20.
20. Romo RD, Wallhagen MI, Yourman L, et al. Perceptions of successful aging among diverse elders with late-life disability. Gerontologist 2013;53(6):939–49.
21. Baltes PB, Baltes MM. Psychological perspectives on successful aging: the model of selective optimization with compensation. In: Baltes PB, Baltes MM, editors. Successful aging: perspectives from the behavioral sciences. Cambridge (England): Cambridge University Press; 1990. p. 1–34.
22. Baltes PB, Freund AM. Human strengths as the orchestration of wisdom and selective optimization with compensation. In: Aspinwall LG, Staudinger UM, editors. A psychology of human strengths: fundamental questions and future directions for a positive psychology. Washington, DC: American Psychological Association; 2003. p. 23–35.
23. Carstensen LL, Fung H, Charles ST. Socioemotional selectivity theory and the regulation of emotion in the second half of life. Motiv Emot 2003;27:103–23.
24. Kahana E, Kahana B. Conceptual and empirical advances in understanding aging well through proactive adaptation. In: Bengtson V, editor. Adulthood and aging: research on continuities and discontinuities. New York: Springer; 1995. p. 18–40.
25. Britton A, Shipley M, Singh-Manoux A, et al. Successful aging: the contribution of early-life and midlife risk factors. J Am Geriatr Soc 2008;56(6):1098–105.

26. Jeste DV, Depp CA, Vahia IV. Successful cognitive and emotional aging. World J Psychiatry 2010;9:78–84.

27. Young Y, Frick KD, Phelan EA. Can successful aging and chronic illness coexist in the same individual? a multidimensional concept of successful aging. J Am Med Dir Assoc 2009;10:87–92.

28. Young Y, Fan MY, Parrish JM, et al. Validation of a novel successful aging construct. J Am Med Dir Assoc 2009;10:314–22.

29. McLaughlin SJ, Jette AM, Connell CM. An examination of healthy aging across a conceptual continuum prevalence estimates, demographic patters, and validity. J Gerontol A Biol Sci Med Sci 2012;67:783–9.

30. Xia X, Chen W, McDermott J, et al. Molecular and phenotypic biomarkers of aging. F1000Res 2017;6:860.

31. Guralnik JM, Ferrucci L, Simonsick EM, et al. Lower-extremity function in persons over the age of 70 years as a predictor of subsequent disability. N Engl J Med 1995;332:556–61.

32. Studenski S, Perera S, Patel K, et al. Gait speed and survival in older adults. JAMA 2011;305:50–8.

33. Vermeulen J, Neyens JC, van Rossum E, et al. Predicting ADL disability in community-dwelling elderly people using physical frailty indicators: a systematic review. BMC Geriatr 2011;11:338.

34. Belsky DW, Moffitt TE, Cohen AA, et al. Eleven telomere, epigenetic clock, and Biomarker-composite quantifications of biological aging: do they measure the same thing? Am J Epidemiol 2018;187(6):1220–30.

35. Neugarten BL. Age groups in American society and the rise of the young-old. Ann Am Acad Polit Soc Sci 1974;415:187–98.

36. Suzman R, Riley MW. Introducing the "oldest old". Milbank Mem Fund Q Health Soc 1985;63:177–86.

37. Beard JR, Officer A, de Carvalho IA, et al. The World report on ageing and health: a policy framework for healthy ageing. Lancet 2016;387(10033):2145–54.

38. Walter LC, Covinsky KE. Cancer screening in elderly patients: a framework for individualized decision making. JAMA 2001;285(21):2750–6.

39. National Prevention Council, US Department of Health and Human Services. Healthy aging in action. Washington, DC: US Department of Health and Human Services; 2016.

40. Nahin RL, Barnes PM, Stussman BJ. Expenditures on complementary health approaches: United States, 2012. Natl Health Stat Report 2016;(95):1–11.

41. Depp CA, Jeste DV. Definitions and predictors of successful aging: a comprehensive review of larger quantitative studies. Am J Geriatr Psychiatry 2006; 14(1):6–20.

42. Louie GH, Ward MM. Socioeconomic and ethnic differences in disease burden and disparities in physical function in older adults. Am J Public Health 2011; 101(7):1322–9.

43. Mühlig-Versen A, Bowen CE, Staudinger UM. Personality plasticity in later adulthood: contextual and personal resources are needed to increase openness to new experiences. Psychol Aging 2012;27(4):855–66.

How Do Geriatric Principles Inform Healthy Aging?

Jennifer D. Muniak, MD[a],*, Paul Mulhausen, MD[b,1]

KEYWORDS

- Healthy aging • Lifestyle medicine • Functional optimization

KEY POINTS

- Geriatricians are well suited and needed to address healthy aging as a core objective of scholarship and advocacy.
- Compression of morbidity, or maintaining a high level of function and vitality throughout the lifespan, requires attention to environmental, social, and structural causes of disease in addition to pathophysiology.
- Several geriatrics principles and approaches translate well to lifestyle medicine, such as aptitude for complex and holistic thinking, appreciation for low technology, high-touch modalities; reliance on high-functioning systems; and focus on person-centered care and functional optimization.

HEALTHY AGING AS A CORE OBJECTIVE FOR GERIATRIC MEDICINE

Since the early days of modern geriatrics, gerontologists have recognized that major differences exist between populations in age-related diseases and age-related physiologic decline.[1] The variability seen in the aging experience across individuals and populations implicated both hereditary and environmental factors.[2] The experience of health over the course of an individual's aging experience was found to depend on both the genetics and the lifestyle of the individual.[3] This variability and the determinants of this variability led to a remarkable insight—not everything declines with age. Some physiologic changes can be slowed or reversed and some of the adverse impacts of age-related diseases could be postponed or prevented.[4] Armed with these insights and recognizing that chronic illness had become responsible for most death and disability, James Fries introduced the compression of morbidity theory,[5] in which the amount of disability can decrease as morbidity is compressed into an ever-shortening span between an increasing age at onset of disability and a fixed maximum

[a] Division of Geriatrics, University of Rochester School of Medicine and Dentistry, Rochester, NY, USA; [b] Iowa Total Care, Iowa City, IA, USA
[1] Present address: 200 Hawkins Drive, Iowa City, IA 52242.
* Corresponding author. Department of Medicine, Highland Hospital, Box 58, 1000 South Avenue, Rochester, NY 14620.
E-mail address: jennifer_muniak@urmc.rochester.edu

Clin Geriatr Med 36 (2020) 559–567
https://doi.org/10.1016/j.cger.2020.06.014
0749-0690/20/© 2020 Elsevier Inc. All rights reserved.

age of death. This vision of aging conceptualized the potential postponement of chronic illness into the extremes of old age. The potential to square the curve is at the root of many visions for a healthy aging experience.

Geriatric medicine has long promoted healthy aging measures to postpone chronic illness, maintain vigor, and slow social involution and achieve the goals implied by the compression of morbidity theory—a central philosophic tenet. But, as noted in a recent article by Friedman and colleagues,[6] both clinical and scholarly attention paid to healthy aging have been outpaced by an interest in frailty. This has been driven largely by the demographic realities of an aging population[7] and the need for a scarce supply of geriatricians to focus their clinical expertise on a high-need population.[8] Typical priority subsets for geriatricians' care include the oldest old (aged 85 and above), complex biomedical and psychosocial situations, those with geriatric syndromes, those who are frail, those who require palliative or end-of-life care, and those who require skilled facilities.[9] Although appropriate and necessary to direct clinical efforts to the most frail and multimorbid, geriatricians possess important expertise that can be brought to bear on the health of all older adults. Measures that educate future patients and incentivize them to lead healthy lifestyles much earlier in life are necessary ingredients for the healthy aging revolution at the individual and societal levels promised by the compression of morbidity theory.

Unfortunately, this is an unprecedented time in history, with ominous trends in poor lifestyle putting future patients at risk for early onset of chronic diseases and consequent disability and frailty. Moreover, standard models of care in the United States are not optimally designed to keep patients healthy and functional for as long as possible. A substantial shift in medical culture, priorities, and allocation of resources is necessary to support a large-scale, successful, healthy aging trend for aging populations.

Geriatricians are well positioned and needed to take on the challenges of healthy aging, given the embedded priorities, abilities, and cognitive constructs of the field. A new and developing branch of medicine, lifestyle medicine, is 1 mechanism for promoting healthy aging in younger populations. Lifestyle medicine is an evidence-based approach to preventing, treating, and even reversing diseases by replacing unhealthy behaviors with positive ones, namely in 6 domains: healthful eating of a whole, plant-based diet; avoiding risky substances; improving sleep; forming and maintaining relationships; developing strategies to manage stress; and increasing physical activity.[10] Many geriatrics principles and approaches to patient care also are applicable to lifestyle medicine. This synergy should further empower geriatricians to take up the mantle of healthy aging for patients.

CONCEPTUAL AND CONTENT OVERLAP BETWEEN GERIATRICS AND LIFESTYLE MEDICINE
APTITUDE FOR COMPLEXITY AND HOLISTIC THINKING

"Geriatricians are complexivists, with the cognitive skills to analyze complex health issues and establish priorities consistent with patient goals and knowledge of models of care delivery that match the healthcare needs of patients," say esteemed geriatricians Fried and Hall[11] in a 2008 editorial. Geriatricians, through training and natural inclination, consider not only many concurrent disease processes but also how a patient is interacting within family systems, other community institutions, function (and level of disability), geriatric syndromes, goals, and values (**Fig. 1**). The challenge and art of balancing multiple priorities and delivering sound counsel to patients are what draw many geriatricians to the field.

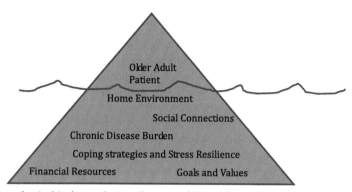

Fig. 1. Metaphorical iceberg, that is, the care of the older adult patient.

Geriatricians as complexivists alternatively can be viewed as holistic practitioners of medicine, in that they work to comprehend of the many parts of a patient's life as intimately interconnected and explicable only by reference to the whole. This is in contrast to a reductionist model, in which complex phenomena are explained by way of a collection of simpler processes. Some health care practitioners may be informed by reductionist principles, and this is appropriate in times when a single solution is needed for a discrete problem, such as surgery to remove an inflamed appendix or placement of a pacemaker to deliver regularly timed electrical impulses to the heart. Reductionist thinking is attractive because of its simplicity and speed; however, when applied inappropriately, a reductionist approach has the potential to miss crucial details and interactions and even cause harm.

The fields of both geriatrics and lifestyle medicine are confronted primarily by problems that fail reductionist thinking. Practitioners of these fields need to embrace the complex, overlapping, messy, and always changing nature of patients' lives. When they do, they can reach the patients and find tangible ways to help them. For example, a geriatrician may be treating an individual with advanced coronary disease, severe generalized anxiety, gait instability, food insecurity, and vision impairment. Managing this patient takes an expertise of the individual conditions on their own, the interactions between geriatrician and patient, and how the geriatrician interacts with the patient's resources (personal, health care, and community) and values. Similarly, a practitioner of lifestyle medicine may be treating an individual trying to make positive behavior changes in the setting of severe obesity, addiction to alcohol, a demanding work environment with low levels of autonomy and competence, and ingrained familial habits of unhealthy food choices. In both of these scenarios, one with a geriatric patient and one with a lifestyle medicine patient, every component of the story is important and contributes to a richer understanding of a patient's circumstances. Taking the time to understand more fully also illuminates a path forward as geriatricians guide patients toward solutions that, although not silver bullets, can be life altering for the better.

LOW-TECH, HIGH-TOUCH APPROACH

Low-tech, high-touch medicine is that which heals by way of time and attention paid to the patient. Integral to the approach is the development of a therapeutic alliance, with a shared understanding of a patient's values and outlook for the patients' health. Specific treatment modalities tout a low-tech, high touch approach and confer additional benefit based on specialized content. These include but are not limited to physical, occupational, speech, cognitive behavioral, and psychodynamic therapy; support groups; dietary counseling; and nursing care.

Such approaches generally are low risk and useful for longitudinal gain. Using them in conjunction with, or in place of, riskier therapies may have downstream benefits of reducing polypharmacy and simplifying a treatment plan. Minimizing high risk therapies is of critical importance for older adult patients who are, as a group, highly vulnerable to risks of other treatment modalities, including medications, because of the following:

- High toxicity: as people age, they have higher inherent risk of medication toxicity compared with younger counterparts: their metabolism of medications slows, less total body water and more fat can make medications last longer in the system.
- Interactions, side effects: older patients are prone to polypharmacy, typically defined as being on many medications or on any unnecessary medications. Polypharmacy can increase the risk of medication interactions and side effects.
- Complexity and decreased adherence: as the medication list grows longer, costs and complexity rise. Patients often lose the ability and desire to adhere to the regimen prescribed and may give up on taking their medication alogether.[12] Simplifying the medication list can have an immense good for patient understanding the rationale and following through with treatment.
- Prescribing cascade: every medication carries a risk of side effects, and with those side effects the potential for the *prescribing cascade*, that is, prescribing medications to treat side effects of other medications. This is a vicious cycle that is difficult to stop. The ideal way to stop the prescribing cascade is to prevent it from starting, by prescribing as few medications as possible.

Low-tech, high-touch approaches can be difficult to sell to patients given that they often require a longitudinal commitment and can be of variable quality, availability, and affordability. Such approaches, however, often are at the core of transformative and sustainable benefits for patients across a variety of settings. For example, older adults suffering from the cognitive and behavioral symptoms are vulnerable to over-reliance on the use of medications that are advertised direct to consumers; when well-executed psychosocial interventions may be just as or more effective.[13]

In a similar fashion to the field of geriatrics, the field of lifestyle medicine places great emphasis on low-tech, high-touch solutions that empower the individual to combat illness and optimize function in a sustainable way. Therefore, at a fundamental level, geriatricians are equipped in this way to help patients make positive lifestyle changes and improve their outlook for healthy aging. Although younger and/or more functional patients may not have the same vulnerability to medications and other high-risk treatment modalities, they too can benefit from a low-tech, high-touch approach to their care. Consider the following case as an illustration.

Patient Case

Consider the story of a fictitious patient, Mr X. He is a 75-year-old man with type 2 diabetes mellitus who is active and independent with all activities of daily living (ADLs) and instrumental ADLs (IADLs). He has had a diagnosis of diabetes for 10 years, since age 65. Since then, he has successfully controlled his blood glucose levels using metformin as a single agent. His hemoglobin A_{1C}, however, is now 8.5, and his physician recommends treatment with insulin because his pancreatic insulin production is inadequate in the face of pancreatic senescence and progressive insulin resistance caused by consuming high loads of glucose and fat.

Mr X is resistant to start insulin due to the cost and inconvenience of daily injections. He, therefore, is prescribed a whole-food, plant-based diet as well as a regimen of daily exercise. Over the next 6 months, his hemoglobin A_{1C} drops from 8.5 to 7, which is within the goal for a patient of his health status, goals, and prognosis.[14] He successfully avoids using insulin.

Despite success in curing or controlling a disease process with lifestyle, a patient such as Mr X may have a disease like diabetes resurface. This is common particularly in older adults who continue to lose physiologic reserve and organ function through the life span. Additionally, older adults may acquire other health problems that reduce their ability to fully participate in healthy lifestyle, such as

- Cognitive impairment
- Loss of ADLs/IADLs and associated autonomy (in particular, driving, meal preparation, and moving to a facility)
- Social isolation
- Degenerative neurologic or musculoskeletal conditions that limit mobility

In such scenarios, it can seem as though lifestyle interventions have failed. Clinicians are needed precisely in these moments to bring additional perspective to the discussion:

- Healthy lifestyle interventions can reduce the total dosage of medication needed for a given medical problem (if not eliminate the need all-together). Often, side effects are dose dependent.
- Lifestyle interventions undertaken earlier in life may delay the onset of disease and thus have the potential to significantly reduce total exposure to the disease process and dependence upon medications or other treatments. For example, in hypertension, an older adult with a mild to moderate form of the condition actually can be considered a good sign for prognosis[15] and may require less intensive treatment[16] versus no medical treatment.

APPRECIATION OF ENVIRONMENTAL AND STRUCTURAL FORCES ON OUTCOMES

Traditionally, clinical practice has focused on determinants of disease at a level proximal to the patient based in pathophysiology, whereas public health has focused more on distal causes of disease to populations that are at an environmental or systems level. Esteemed physician and medical anthropologist Paul Farmer calls on clinicians to integrate a more holistic view of disease determinants and not ignore the structural and more distal causes of disease. Farmer and colleagues[17] describe a phenomenon of "structural violence," which can exert harm to individuals and populations through social arrangements that are embedded in political and economic organizations. Their public health work keeps them in close touch with system forces that created barriers to care for populations, particularly those with disease processes, such as HIV. By implementing comprehensive structural interventions to vulnerable populations, their organization was able to achieve impressive patient outcomes.[17]

Geriatricians inherently are attuned to the value of high-functioning systems in the well-being of older adult patients. When considering the systems of a family unit, care facility personnel, or community health partners, geriatricians understand that older adults (particularly those with high levels of medical complexity and dependency) require high-functioning systems to keep them healthy. They also appreciate how low levels of support or frankly unsafe environments can lead to harm.

Many innovative care models are in place for older patients that place a premium value upon infrastructure. One such program is the Program of All-Inclusive Care for the Elderly (PACE), which provides comprehensive health services for those aged 55 and above who are considered nursing home eligible by their state's Medicaid program yet remain in their homes through creative, coordinated deployment of health care resources. Although the population of PACE is very frail and medically complex, the program helps keep its participants in their homes with a combination of regular medical care, structured day programs and social events, and individualized deployment of monies to treat chronic medical conditions. The PACE program generally has showed positive patient satisfaction, reduction in institutional care, and controlled utilization of medical services as well as cost savings to the Medicare and Medicaid programs.[18]

As American health care continues through a period of unprecedented change in combination with an aging baby boomer population, there is a greater need than ever to have universally available high-functioning health systems for older adults. The framework of an Age-Friendly Health System has emerged as a model for universal adoption by health systems to implement high-quality, cost-effective care models for geriatric patients. The model is based around consistently assessing and acting on 4 domains of health for the older adult, described as the 4 Ms: medications, mobility, mind/mentation, and matters to the older adult (honoring choice and implementing care within the context of a patient's value system).[19] The simplicity of this model lends well to adaptation in a variety of health care settings and institutional cultures.

Older adults also need broader environmental shifts that are explicitly designed to help them. The now well-described Blue Zones are composed of 5 areas of the world with unusually high rates of quality longevity, originally described by Buettner[20]: Loma Linda, California; Nicoya, Costa Rica; Sardinia, Italy; Ikaria, Greece; and Okinawa, Japan. Buettner has isolated 9 evidence-based common denominators of longevity associated with the Blue Zones:

- Move naturally—aim for consistent activity throughout the day.
- Purpose—have a reason to wake up in the morning.
- Downshift—stress may be unavoidable, but Blue Zones residents have regular means of self-care.
- The 80% rule—otherwise put, mindful consumption of food and drink, without trying to be full at the end of the meal. This can mean the difference between weight maintenance and gaining.
- Plant slant—beans, including fava, black, soy, and lentils, are the cornerstone of most centenarian diets. Meat is consumed less often and, by subsets of the Adventists in Loma Linda, not at all.
- Wine at 5:00 PM—people in all Blue Zones (except Adventists) drink alcohol moderately and regularly.
- Belong—most interviewed centenarians had an active faith community. Denomination did not seem to matter.
- Loved ones first—successful centenarians in the Blue Zones put their families first, meaning keeping aging parents and grandparents nearby or in the home, committing to a life partner, and investing in their children with time and love.
- Right tribe—having a social circle is important for many health outcomes, including longevity. Health behaviors are contagious!

Blue Zones pilot projects have transposed the critical concepts from the original Blue Zones to other communities with success. Through changes to infrastructure and policy changes that promoted health and wellness, participants in Albert Lea, Montana, mounted impressive improvements to their life spans (+2.9 years), weight loss, a drop in tobacco usage, and improvement in physical activity.[21] Health-promoting environments can be manufactured at small large and at large scale and doing so is within the skill set of all in health care.

FOCUS ON PERSON-CENTERED TREATMENT AND FUNCTIONAL OPTIMIZATION

Those in geriatrics are highly attuned toward promoting highest quality of life and function for their patients, perhaps because attaining these positive outcomes cannot be taken for granted in the setting of escalating chronic disease burden and advancing age. Flexible and creative person-centered strategies are needed to prioritize goals and values. Patients with the same disease process can choose wildly divergent paths based on several factors, with common themes being

- Tolerance for the burdens of medical care
- Financial resources
- Religious and/or cultural customs
- Family and other social supports
- Patient perception of a treatment's risks and benefits

Because each patient's algorithm is unique, geriatricians are skilled in eliciting motivations and values, thus caring for patients in a collaborative, person-centered way.

Patient circumstances also dictate how to best care for them and need to be considered alongside goals and values. Such considerations for geriatricians often include physical, cognitive, and psychiatric functions; comorbid conditions; prognosis; and social support. Functional optimization, treatment, and prevention look very different for a patient with advanced dementia in a nursing home compared with an independent older adult living in the community. Both individuals deserve thoughtful clinicians, however, who meet them where they are and work with them to optimize their function in a patient-centered way.

Similarly, promotion of healthy lifestyle can be conceptualized as a person-centered process that transcends age and abilities. It is a process that begins by accepting patients where they are and guides them to meaningful outcomes, utilizing their motivations, values, and supports as tools in the process. **Table 1** is an example of how the same 3 goals can have drastically different motivations for different hypothetical patients.

Making positive lifestyle changes is difficult, and at any point in time there likely is a limit to what can be achieved based on an individual's function and resources. For any number of reasons, it may not be possible for a patient to make a complete, sustained behavior change, such as abstinence from addictive substances, adoption of a consistently healthful diet, achieving a high fitness level, and so forth.

Geriatricians are particularly well suited to guide patients in a nuanced and compassionate way in such moments that lend themselves so easily to shame, self-doubt, and all-or-none thinking. Perhaps they are resilient to all-or-none thinking because the care of older adults requires appreciating the immense impact that can come from relatively small changes in treatment. For example, a patient may be able to control incontinence with a scheduled toileting program or may feel less fatigue with a modest dose reduction of a psychotropic medication. Celebrating these victories with patients is intensely gratifying and would be lost if geriatricians were blind to what can be achieved with incremental adjustments. Translating this perspective to the world of lifestyle medicine and healthy aging similarly can help geriatricians celebrate the incremental victories that come from cutting down on alcohol or tobacco usage, reducing processed foods, or starting a physical activity routine.

Table 1
Goals and motivations

Goal	Motivation for Individual A—20 y	Motivation for Individual B—40 y	Motivation for Individual C—60 y
Quit smoking	I want more disposable income.	I want a different fate than my father, who just died of lung cancer.	I want better exercise tolerance.
Improve health content of diet	I want to have less acne and lose weight.	I want to model appropriate eating behaviors to my children.	I want to avoid a second heart attack.
Increase fitness	I want to participate in competitive sports.	I want to have more energy during the day.	I want to be independent with ADLs for as long as possible.

DISCLOSURE

Dr. Jennifer D. Muniak have received grant funding by Health Resources Services Administration (HRSA) as an awardee of the Geriatrics Academic Career Award, award number: 5 K01 HP33458-02-00.

REFERENCES

1. Lindeman RD, Tobin J, Shock NW. Longitudinal studies in the rate of decline in renal function with age. J Am Geriatr Soc 1985;33(4):278–85.
2. Goldstein S. The biology of aging. N Engl J Med 1971;285:1120–9.
3. Sobel H. Ageing and age-associated disease. Lancet 1970;2(7684):1191–2.
4. Rowe JW, Kahn RL. Human aging: usual and successful. Science 1987;237(4811):143–9.
5. Fries JF. Aging, Natural Death, and the Compression of Morbidity. New England Journal of Medicine 1980;303(3):130–5.
6. Friedman S, Shah K, Hall W. Failing to focus on healthy aging: a frailty of our discipline? J Am Geriatr Soc 2015;63(7):1459–62.
7. Schneider EL, Brody JA. Aging, natural death, and the compression of morbidity: another view. N Engl J Med 1983;3019(14):854–6.
8. Besdine R, Boult C, Brangman S, et al. Caring for older Americans: the future of geriatric medicine. J Am Geriatr Soc 2005;53(6 Suppl):S245–56.
9. Fried LP, Hall WJ. Leading on behalf of an aging society. J Am Geriatr Soc 2008;56:1791–5.
10. Available at: https://lifestylemedicine.org/What-is-Lifestyle-Medicine Accessed December 27, 2019.
11. Editorial: leading on behalf of an aging society. - NCBI. Available at: https://www.ncbi.nlm.nih.gov/pubmed/19054197. Accessed October 4, 2019.
12. Medication non-adherence among elderly patients newly. Available at: https://www.ncbi.nlm.nih.gov/pubmed/24604085. Accessed November 17, 2019.
13. Morley JE. Managing persons with dementia in the nursing home: high touch trumps high tech. J Am Med Dir Assoc 2008;9(3):139–46.
14. American Geriatrics Society | choosing wisely. Available at: https://www.choosingwisely.org/societies/american-geriatrics-society/. Accessed November 1, 2019.

15. Embracing complexity: a consideration of hypertension ... - NCBI. Available at: https://www.ncbi.nlm.nih.gov/pubmed/12865483. Accessed November 7, 2019.

16. Lower blood pressure during antihypertensive treatment is associated. 2018. Available at: https://www.ncbi.nlm.nih.gov/pubmed/29741555. Accessed November 7, 2019.

17. Farmer PE, Nizeye B, Stulac S, et al. Structural violence and clinical medicine. PLoS Med 2006;3(10):e449.

18. Eng C, Pedulla J, Eleazer GP, et al. Program of all-inclusive care for the elderly (PACE): an innovative model of integrated geriatric care and financing. J Am Geriatr Soc 1997;45:223–32.

19. Fulmer T, Mate KS, Berman A. The age-friendly health system imperative. J Am Geriatr Soc 2018;66(1):22–4.

20. Blue zones - NCBI. 2016. Available at: https://www.ncbi.nlm.nih.gov/pmc/articles/PMC6125071/. Accessed November 18, 2019.

21. Available at: https://www.ruralhealthinfo.org/project-examples/812 Accessed December 27, 2019

Multimorbidity, Function, and Cognition in Aging

Sindhuja Kadambi, MD[a],*, Maya Abdallah, MD[b], Kah Poh Loh, MBBCh[a]

KEYWORDS

- Multimorbidity • Comorbidity • Aging • Concurrent disease • Cumulative effect

KEY POINTS

- Multimorbidity is the co-occurrence of 2 or more diseases or conditions in the same individual.
- Biological, psychological, behavioral, socioeconomic, and environmental factors all play a role in multimorbidity.
- Multimorbidity is associated with decreased physical functioning, cognitive functioning, quality of life, and increased mortality.
- Multimorbidity is a global health challenge that is associated with increased health care use.

DEFINING COMORBIDITY AND MULTIMORBIDITY

Comorbidity and multimorbidity are important health factors that require complex medical management and are associated with worse health outcomes and increased health care costs. *Comorbidity* is defined as the occurrence of more than 1 disease or age-related health condition in an individual. *Multimorbidity* is broadly defined as the co-occurrence of 2 or more diseases or conditions in the same individual.[1,2] However, simply counting the number of illnesses does not fully capture the extent of their impact on a patient's health and number alone cannot be used alone to examine the impact of multimorbidity on health care barriers, use, and costs. Currently, there exists no consensus on how to the term "multimorbidity" should be operationalized and its definition has varied based on the context in which it is used, that is, for clinical care, epidemiologic research, or health service planning.

The 3 major operational definitions of multimorbidity that exist in literature are[3]:

1. Two or more concurrent diseases in the same individual, without considering effect of disease on function;

[a] Department of Hematology/Oncology, University of Rochester, 601 Elmwood Drive, Rochester, NY 14642, USA; [b] Department of Medicine, Baystate Health, Springfield, MA 01199, USA
* Corresponding author.
E-mail address: sindhuja_kadambi@urmc.rochester.edu
Twitter: @kgsindhu (S.K.)

Clin Geriatr Med 36 (2020) 569–584
https://doi.org/10.1016/j.cger.2020.06.002
geriatric.theclinics.com

2. Cumulative indices such as the Charlson Comorbidity Index (CCI)[4] that incorporate both number and severity of concurrent diseases; and
3. The presence of not only concurrent diseases, but also symptoms and impairments in physical and cognitive function.

Multimorbidity is thought to differ from comorbidity in that it examines overall health issues, whereas comorbidity is considered in the relation to an index disease.

Measuring Multimorbidity

Measuring multimorbidity is important for determining its impact on individuals and outcomes. However, the absence of a clear definition for multimorbidity contributes to the lack of standardized methods to measure it. Measurements are complex because they depend on the population studied, outcome of interest (ie, mortality vs disability) and the context in which it is used (ie, clinical practice vs outcomes research). For the time being, these measures are largely used in research studies and have not been applied in clinical practice.

The most extensively studied method is the CCI, which calculates disease severity by mortality risk. The CCI, developed in 1987, includes 19 conditions with each condition weighted based on estimated 1-year mortality hazard ratio from a Cox proportional hazards model and generates a total comorbidity score by summing the weighted conditions (**Table 1**).[4] It has been reliably shown to predict mortality across a variety of populations, including but not limited to older adults, patients with cancer,

Table 1
Comorbidities and assigned scores for the CCI

Comorbidity	Score
Prior myocardial infarction	1
Congestive heart failure	1
Peripheral vascular disease	1
Cerebrovascular disease	1
Dementia	1
Chronic pulmonary disease	1
Rheumatologic disease	1
Peptic ulcer disease	1
Mild liver disease	1
Diabetes	1
Cerebrovascular (hemiplegia) event	2
Moderate-to-severe renal disease	2
Diabetes with chronic complications	2
Cancer without metastases	2
Leukemia	2
Lymphoma	2
Moderate to severe liver disease	3
Metastatic solid tumor	6
AIDS	6

Adapted from Quan H, Li B, Couris CM, et al. Updating and validating the Charlson comorbidity index and score for risk adjustment in hospital discharge abstracts using data from 6 countries. Am J Epidemiol. 2011;173(6):678; with permission.

heart disease, and end-stage renal disease, as well as in patients undergoing surgical procedures.[5] It has also been shown to be associated with disability, hospital length of stay and hospital readmissions.

The Cumulative Illness Rating Scale is another commonly used scale.[6] It was developed in 1968 to assess physical impairment and differs from the CCI in that it assesses the severity of impairment in 13 areas grouped by body systems rather than the presence of specific illnesses. It heavily depends on clinical judgment (**Table 2**). Similar to the CCI, it has been shown to be reliable in a variety of different clinical contexts and it has been shown to predict a variety of outcomes such as morbidity, health outcomes, and health care use.[7,8]

Wei and colleagues[9,10] recently developed and validated a multimorbidity weighted index (MWI) for community-dwelling adults aged 54 to 89 years that combines both the presence of chronic conditions as well as their impact. Their index weighs chronic conditions to their impact on the Short Form-36 physical functioning scale, a validated instrument used to assess health-related quality of life. It was found to accurately predict mortality and outperformed the CCI, even though the MWI is weighted to physical functioning and the CCI is weighted to mortality. This patient-centered, quantitative measure of multimorbidity is proposed as a readily feasible tool for research and ambulatory practice, requiring only self-reported information on past medical history and impact on function. An online calculator for the MWI has been developed and is publicly available through the Division of Geriatrics at the University of California San Francisco (**Box 1**).[11]

Demographics of Adults with Comorbidity/Multimorbidity

Overall life expectancy is improving worldwide, with the World Health Organization estimating the mean age of 72 years in more than 60 countries. The chronic medical conditions increases with age (**Fig. 1**), the prevalence of multimorbidity is also expected to increase.[12,13]

Table 2	
Diseases and scoring system for cumulative illness rating scale for geriatrics	
Organ-System Categories	**Rating Strategy**
1. Heart	0 – No problem
2. Vascular	1 – Current mild problem or past significant problem
3. Hematopoietic	2 – Moderate disability or morbidity/requires
4. Respiratory	"first-line" therapy
5. Eyes, ears, nose, throat and larynx	3 – Severe/constant significant difficulty/ "uncontrollable" chronic problems
6. Upper gastrointestinal tract	4 – Extremely severe/immediate treatment required/
7. Lower gastrointestinal tract	end organ failure/severe impairment of function
8. Liver	
9. Renal	
10. Genitourinary	
11. Musculoskeletal/integument	
12. Neurologic	
13. Endocrine/metabolic and breast	
14. Psychiatric illness	

From Miller MD, Paradis CF, Houck PR, et al. Rating chronic medical illness burden in geropsychiatric practice and research: Application of the Cumulative Illness Rating Scale. Psychiatry Res. 1992;41(3):237-248; with permission.

Box 1

Case example calculating functional decline and mortality using the MWI

Community-dwelling man aged 65 years with chronic lung disease (chronic obstructive lung disease), hypertension, and diabetes.

Chronic Disease or Condition	Multimorbidity-Weighted Index (MWI) Weighting
Chronic lung disease (chronic obstructive lung disease)	4.32
Hypertension	1.53
Diabetes	2.67
Total MWI score	8.52

His total MWI score is 8.52: 1 point on MWI = 3 years of additional aging (physical functioning decline) over 8 years in the same person.

This translates to 25.56 years of additional aging over the course of 8 years.

His 10-year all-cause mortality risk is 34.1%.

Calculated using https://eprognosis.ucsf.edu/mwi.php, accessed March 18, 2020. Summary of all conditions and weights can be found in Wei MY, Mukamal KJ. Multimorbidity, mortality, and long-term physical functioning in 3 prospective cohorts of community-dwelling adults. Am J Epidemiol 2018;187:103–112.

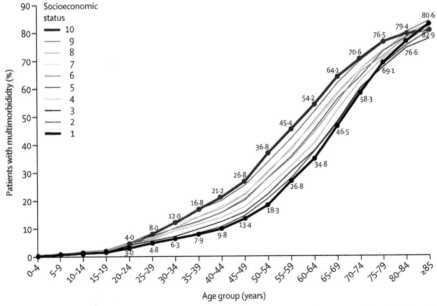

Fig. 1. Prevalence of multimorbidity by age and socioeconomic status. (Reprinted with permission from Elsevier. From Barnett K et al. Epidemiology of multimorbidity and implications for health care, research, and medical education: a cross-sectional study. The Lancet. 2012;380(9836):39.)

Estimating the prevalence of multimorbidity is important in determining population disease burden, resources for interventions, and health care costs, but estimates can vary based on definition and measure of multimorbidity use. In a systemic review and meta-analysis, Nguyen and colleagues[14] found that although there were regional variations, the global prevalence of multimorbidity was 33.1% (95% confidence interval [CI], 30.0%–36.3%). The prevalence of multimorbidity is increasing over time in part owing to improved survival, an aging population, and earlier and improved detection of diseases, as well as changing lifestyle factors.[15] In the United States, a 2010 National Health Interview Survey, found that 26% of adults had 2 or more chronic conditions, increased from 21.8% in 2001.[16] Studies have also shown the following patterns of prevalence of multimorbidity[17,18]:

- Prevalence of multimorbidity increases with age. More than 50% of individuals 65 and over have multimorbidity. The highest prevalence in the "oldest old" 85 and over group.
- Women have greater prevalence of multimorbidity than men.
- Prevalence varies by race/ethnicity. In the US population, prevalence was highest among American Indian/Alaska native, followed by non-Hispanic white and non-Hispanic black adults and lowest in Hispanic and Asian adults.
- Multimorbidity is more prevalent in people with mental health disorders.

Effect of Socioeconomic Status on Prevalence

There are differences in the prevalence of multimorbidity based on socioeconomic status (see **Fig. 1**). In a cross-sectional study of self-reported multimorbidity of 5010 adults 18 years and older in Canada, the prevalence of multimorbidity was higher in individuals with lower income (11.6% in those earing >100,000 vs 32.5% in those earing <30,000; odds ratio, 2.39; 95% CI, 1.72–3.33; $P = .041$) and in those with less education (15.2% in those with a university-level education vs 20.8% in those with high school education; odds ratio, 1.11; 95% CI, 0.86–1.42, $P = .007$).[17] In a cross-sectional study in Scotland, compared with age-matched controls, multimorbidity occurred 10 to 15 years earlier in adults living in deprived areas and socioeconomic deprivation was associated with more physical and mental health disorders (11%; 95% CI, 10.9%–11.2% in the most deprived areas vs 5.9%; 95% CI, 5.8%–6.0% in the least deprived areas).[8] Certain illnesses, including chronic obstructive pulmonary disease, coronary heart disease, diabetes, cancer, depression, and pain disorders, were more common in lower income areas, whereas others such as dementia and atrial fibrillation were more common in higher income areas.

MECHANISM OF DISEASE AND DISABILITY
Effects of Lifestyle Factors

There are complex interactions between biological, psychological, behavioral, socioeconomic, and environmental factors that result in multimorbidity, accelerate aging, and cause decline. Lifestyle factors that predispose individuals to multimorbidity include obesity, lack of physical activity, tobacco and excess alcohol use, and a diet low in fruit and vegetables.[19–22] The overall risk of developing multimorbidity from these factors may depend on specific combinations and additive effects of individual factors.[19,22] In a large study of older adults, although physical inactivity was the only variable independently associated with increased risk of multimorbidity, a combination of 2, 3, and 4 or more unhealthy lifestyle factors (inactivity, smoking, alcohol consumption, fruit and vegetable consumption, and body mass index [BMI]) significantly increased multimorbidity compared with none from 42% to 116%.[19]

Physical inactivity

Physical activity has been shown to have important effects on physical and mental well-being (**Fig. 2**).[23] It can modify the effects of chronic conditions and improve outcomes in a variety of conditions, as well as decrease disability, morbidity, and mortality. In addition to its benefits on cardiovascular and metabolic conditions, physical activity has been shown to prevent cognitive decline and decreases the risk of developing dementia.[24,25] The effects of physical activity on health outcomes are thought to be due to its effects on regulating body weight and its effects on decreasing insulin resistance, hypertension, dyslipidemia, and inflammation.[26] It seems to have a protective effect on neurodegeneration and psychological health by causing structural and

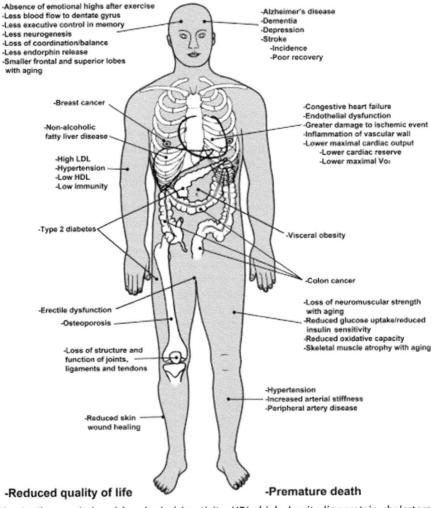

Fig. 2. Changes induced by physical inactivity. HDL, high-density lipoprotein cholesterol; LDL, low-density lipoprotein cholesterol. (*From* Booth FW and Laye MJ. Lack of adequate appreciation of physical exercise's complexities can pre-empt appropriate design and interpretation in scientific discovery. J Physiol. 2009;587(23):5531; with permission.)

functional changes, such as increasing cerebral vascular blood flow and increasing neuroplasticity.[25–27]

Studies on the effects of physical activity on multimorbidity as a whole, however, have been mixed. Studies of older adults have generally found that active older adults benefit from increased activity and have fewer comorbid conditions and lower odds ratio for multimorbidity than nonactive older adults.[28,29] This benefit was found to be true especially in regard to the cardiovascular and metabolic disease cluster.[29] However, a study of younger patients, which did not include older adults over the age of 69, did not show this benefit.[30] Although it is difficult to compare these studies because they used different physical activity assessments, the studies overall seem to suggest there may be age and gender differences in the effects of physical activity on multimorbidity, which need to be elucidated further.

Nutrition
High-calorie diets rich in saturated fats and cholesterol have been shown to be associated with metabolic dysregulation, increased oxidative stress, and increased inflammation, which are all risk factors for obesity, cardiovascular disease, metabolic disorders, arthritis, and various cancers.[31] There are limited studies, however, on the effects of nutrition on multimorbidity. A cross-sectional study found that individuals with a high consumption of a "meat and potatoes" diet had a greater likelihood of cardiometabolic morbidity, with obesity as a likely intermediate step.[32] Similarly, sugar-sweetened beverages have also been associated obesity, cardiovascular disease, and metabolic syndromes. An Australian study found that drinking more than 0.5 L of soft drinks per day versus not drinking any soft drinks increased risk of multimorbidity, and the risk was greater for women than for men.[33] A cohort study of Chinese adults, based on a 3-day weighted food record, found that fruit, vegetable, whole grain, and fiber consumption was greater in healthier individuals.[21]

Obesity
Obesity, which is closely linked to poor nutrition and physical inactivity, is strongly associated with increased inflammation, metabolic derangements, and decrease in physical function, all of which are shared risk factors for cardiovascular and noncardiovascular disease.[34] In a large pooled analysis of 120,813 adults in the United States and Europe, Kivimäki and colleagues[35] found that cardiometabolic multimorbidity, which is defined as the coexistence of more than 1 of type 2 diabetes, coronary artery disease, and stroke, increases with obesity. Compared with individuals with a healthy BMI (20–24.9 kg/m^2), overweight people (BMI of 25–29.9 kg/m^2) had twice the risk, and severely obese people (BMI of $\geq$35 kg/m^2) had 10 times the risk of cardiometabolic multimorbidity. This pattern was similar across age, gender, and ethnicities.

Tobacco and alcohol use
Tobacco and alcohol use, which frequently occur in conjunction with psychiatric comorbidities, are similarly associated with multimorbidity.[36,37] Cigarette smoking is a major risk factor for diseases in all organ systems, including but not limited to cardiovascular and pulmonary disease and cancer.[38] Both a longer duration and a greater intensity of smoking (amount of tobacco smoked per day) are associated with an increased risk of tobacco-related diseases.

Although low levels of alcohol use may have protective effects on heart disease and diabetes, the average volume alcohol consumption is associated with increased risk of multiple diseases, including liver cirrhosis, 8 different cancers, and cardiovascular outcomes such as hypertension and stroke.[39] A recent study showed that alcohol use by men may result in a 3 times higher health loss than by women.[40]

Common Pathways to Chronic Disease

Many of the factors involved in multimorbidity seem to share similar biology pathways (**Fig. 3**).[41] Studies suggest that certain mechanisms related to oxidative stress and chronic inflammation that result in cellular senescence, impaired cell signaling, and cell death are involved.

Role of oxidative stress

Oxidative stress occurs when there is an imbalance in the formation of reactive oxygen species (ROS), which are toxic metabolic byproducts and molecules (antioxidants) that are protective against injury by these free radicals. ROS include superoxide anion ($\bullet O_2^-$), hydroxyl radical ($\bullet OH$), singlet oxygen ($^1O_2$), hydrogen peroxide (H_2O_2), and hypochlorous acid (HOCl). They are unstable molecules because of unpaired electrons and have the capacity to produce damaging free radical chain reactions.[42] ROS are endogenously produced as byproducts of oxygen metabolism. They can be increased in various inflammatory processes, including infections and ischemic injuries. They are also produced by environmental exposures such as UV radiation, cigarette smoking, and alcohol consumption. ROS are removed by enzymatic antioxidants such as such as superoxide dismutase, catalase, and peroxidase, as well as nonenzymatic antioxidants such as vitamin E, β-carotene, and coenzyme Q.[42] At normal levels, ROS have important roles in cellular function and tissue homeostasis. Overproduction of ROS results in alteration of cellular processes and tissue damage. Oxidative stress has been linked to the pathogenesis of aging and disease in every organ, including, but not limited to cancer, cardiovascular disease, diabetes mellitus, respiratory disease, gastrointestinal disorders, and neurodegenerative diseases.[43]

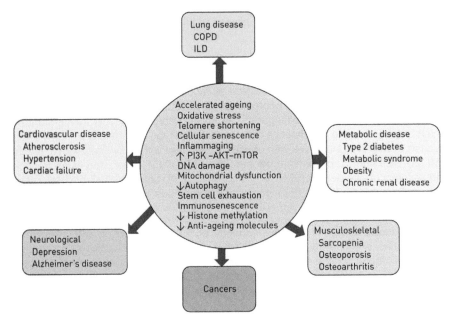

Fig. 3. Biological mechanisms of multimorbidity. COPD, chronic obstructive pulmonary disease; ILD, interstitial lung disease; mTOR, mammalian target of rapamycin. (*From* Barnes PJ. Mechanisms of development of multimorbidity in the elderly. Reproduced with permission of the © ERS 2020: European Respiratory Journal 45 (3) 790-806; DOI: 10.1183/09031936.00229714 Published 28 February 2015.)

Role of inflammation

There are numerous studies that suggest that dysregulated inflammation plays a key role in aging and in many chronic illness including cancers, heart disease, diabetes, dementia and mental health disorders.[44,45] The Midlife in the United States study showed using cross-sectional data from 1229 participants with a mean age of 54.5 years, that multimorbidity was associated with inflammation using the markers IL-6, C-reactive protein, and fibrinogen.[46] This study and others have found that not only is inflammation implicated in the incidence of disease, but that inflammation may also be a link between multimorbidity and disability. Levels of inflammatory markers were found to be higher with accumulation of chronic diseases and higher levels of inflammation are associated with greater functional impairment and disability.[46–48] The mechanism by which inflammatory cytokines exert their effects are yet to be fully elucidated, but may be related to their direct effects on muscle catabolism and their effects on age-related changes in body composition. Inflammation may also play a role in health disparities. Studies have shown that socioeconomic factors such as income and education are associated with inflammatory cytokines.[49,50]

Disease Clustering and Synergistic Effects

As a result of the shared risk factors discussed elsewhere in this article, certain diseases cluster together beyond chance. In a systematic study of the prevalence of disease clusters studied in older adults with multimorbidity, 20 disease pairs composed of 12 different diseases were found to occur frequently.[51] Hypertension, coronary artery disease, and diabetes was the most highly prevalent combination. Depression was the most frequently clustered and occurred in conjunction with 8 different diseases. In fact, mental health disorders are frequently found clustered together. Compared with the general population, psychiatric patients have higher age-standardized relative risk for chronic illness, with obesity, hypertension, hyperlipidemia, and diabetes being significantly more prevalent in this population.[52] In addition to lifestyle factors such as substance use as well as treatment-related effects, psychiatric illness in itself seems to be an important risk factor for developing other comorbid conditions, such as coronary heart disease.[53]

The complex interactions between individual conditions seems to have synergistic effects that accelerate aging and cause functional decline (**Fig. 4**). Using self-reported data from 13,232 adults 50 years or older, Koroukian and colleagues[54] demonstrated that the co-occurrence of chronic conditions, functional limitations and/or geriatric syndromes had additive effects on mortality. Adults with co-occurrence of all 3 were 12 times as likely to die within 2 years. Wei and colleagues[55] also demonstrated in their development of the MWI that individual diseases do not have equal weighted effects on physical performance and mortality and that determination of both these outcomes depends on the cumulative effects of chronic disease.

EFFECTS OF MULTIMORBIDITY ON OUTCOMES
Effects of Multimorbidity on Survival

Multimorbidity is associated with many adverse health outcomes in the general older adult population as well as in specific populations (eg, patients with cancer, health failure, diabetes).[56–58] These health outcomes include decreased physical functioning, cognitive functioning, and quality of life, as well as increased health care use and mortality.[59–61] In a population-based cohort study of adults age 78 years and older in Sweden, multimorbidity ($\geq$2 chronic conditions, out of 38 conditions) affected 70.4% of the population and accounted for most deaths (69.3% of total deaths), followed by

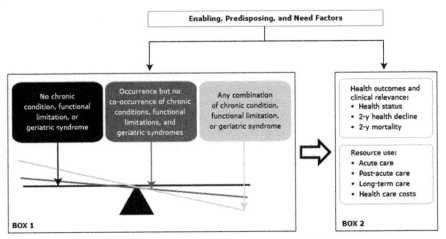

Fig. 4. Cumulative effects of chronic disease, functional limitations, and geriatric syndromes. (*From* Koroukian S, Warner DF, Owusu C, et al. Multimorbidity redefined: prospective health outcomes and the cumulative effect of co-occurring conditions. Prev Chronic Dis. 2015;12:140478.)

cardiovascular (28.0%) and neuropsychiatric diseases (17.0%).[62] It also leads to 7.5 years of life lost, compared with 5.0 and 4.3, respectively, for cardiovascular disease and cancer.[62] Similarly, among community-dwelling adults age 65 years and over enrolled on the National Health and Aging Trends Study in the United States, multimorbidity (or high multisystem morbidity as defined in the study, determined based on Bayesian information criterion) was associated with a greater risk of death.[63]

Effects of Multimorbidity on Physical Functioning

Although survival is important, understanding how multimorbidity affects other patient-centered outcomes such as physical functioning, cognitive functioning, mental health, quality of life, disability, and health care use is also meaningful. Older adults prioritize these outcomes just as much, if not more, than survival.[64,65] They may choose to have a shorter life span (length of life) for a longer health span (length of healthy life). To this end, several population-based cohort studies have evaluated the relationships of multimorbidity with these patient-centered outcomes.[59,66,67] In a longitudinal analysis of adults age 51 and older enrolled on the Health Retirement Study in the United States, those with a higher MWI experienced more decline in physical functioning (measured using the modified Short Form 36).[66] For example, in a 68-year-old man with a stroke and myocardial infarction, his MWI is 5.5, which translates to approximately 5.5 points decrease on the Short Form 36 physical functioning scale, or 16.5 years of additional aging over the course of 8 years. In another cross-sectional analysis of adults age 65 and older enrolled on the National Health and Nutrition Examination Survey in the United States, multimorbidity (≥2 chronic conditions, out of 9 conditions) was associated with an increase in functional limitations.[67] The association was stronger in those age 75 years and older, emphasizing particular vulnerability as one ages.[67]

Effects of Multimorbidity on Cognitive Functioning, Mental Health, and Quality of Life

Like physical functioning, multimorbidity is associated with a decline in cognitive functioning. In the Health Retirement Study, patients with a higher MWI were more likely to experience declines in cognition, specifically global cognition, immediate and delayed recall, and working memory, after 14 years of follow-up.[68] In the Baltimore Longitudinal Study of Aging in the United States, multimorbidity (faster accumulation of 12 chronic diseases ie, $\geq$0.25 diseases per year) was associated with a decrease in performance on verbal fluency tests, measured using standardized neuropsychological batteries.[69] In the Mayo Clinic Study of Aging that included older adults age 70 to 89 years at enrollment, multimorbidity ($\geq$2 chronic conditions, out of 17 conditions and not including dementia) is also linked to mild cognitive impairment and dementia over a median follow-up of 4 years.[70] In terms of mental health and quality of life, patients with a higher MWI had worse mental health-related quality of life.[71] In addition, the risk of suicide mortality was increased (2- to 3-fold higher risk in adults in the highest vs lowest quartile of the MWI).[71] Two systematic reviews and meta-analyses that included 40 and 74 studies also demonstrated that patients with multimorbidity (variable definitions) were more likely to develop depression and reported decreased overall quality of life.[72,73]

Effects of Multimorbidity on Health Care Use and Costs

Hospitalization leads to a decrease in physical and cognitive functioning, increased disability, and poor quality of life.[74,75] Therefore, there are efforts to optimize outpatient management and prevent hospitalization among older adults. Patients with multimorbidity visit their primary care providers and specialists more often, and are more likely to be admitted to the hospital and experience a longer hospital length of stay.[76,77] They are also more likely to require long-term care services.[78] Multimorbidity thereby contributes to higher health care costs and a significant economic burden.[79]

Effects of Multimorbidity on Outcomes in Older Adults with Various Diseases

The negative impact of multimorbidity is consistent across various diseases. For example, among long-term survivors of breast cancer, multimorbidity (assessed on a continuous scale) is associated with reduced physical functioning.[80] Older adults with cancer and multimorbidity also experience higher cancer-specific and overall mortality.[81,82] Among older patients with heart failure, those with multimorbidity (assessed on a continuous scale) reported a lower quality of life.[83] Among middle-aged and older adults with diabetes, its combination with multimorbidity (specifically high depressive symptoms and stroke) also increases the risk of disability.[84] These findings reinforce the impact of multimorbidity on health outcomes in all older adults across all settings.

Effects of Multimorbidity on Outcomes in Middle- and Low-Income Countries

Multimorbidity is not limited to high-income countries. In middle- and low-income countries, multimorbidity is similarly associated with functional limitation, depression, poor self-rated health, and lower quality of life, although the data are more limited in these settings.[85] They are also more susceptible to developing disability.[86] In addition, each unit increase in multimorbidity count increases the cumulative risk of care dependence (needing help from caregivers) by 20%.[87] Mental-related (eg, depression and anxiety) and cognitive-related multimorbidity (eg, dementia) were found to increase the risk of care dependence more than physical multimorbidity.

Together, these studies suggest that multimorbidity is a global health challenge and highlight the need for health care systems to better care for this growing population as well as to better incentivize health care providers to provide the necessary complex care. Interventions are needed to address risk factors for disease, including obesity, physical inactivity and poor nutrition. Interventions are also required to address the effects of multimorbidity on disability once it occurs.

DISCLOSURE

The authors have nothing to disclose.

REFERENCES

1. van den Akker M, Buntinx F, Knottnerus JA. Comorbidity or multimorbidity. Eur J Gen Pract 1996;2(2):65–70.
2. Yancik R, Ershler W, Satariano W, et al. Report of the national institute on aging task force on comorbidity. J Gerontol A Biol Sci Med Sci 2007;62(3):275–80.
3. Marengoni A, Angleman S, Melis R, et al. Aging with multimorbidity: a systematic review of the literature. Ageing Res Rev 2011;10(4):430–9.
4. Charlson ME, Pompei P, Ales KL, et al. A new method of classifying prognostic comorbidity in longitudinal studies: development and validation. J Chronic Dis 1987;40(5):373–83.
5. de Groot V, Beckerman H, Lankhorst GJ, et al. How to measure comorbidity: a critical review of available methods. J Clin Epidemiol 2003;56(3):221–9.
6. Linn BS, Linn MW, Gurel L. Cumulative illness rating scale. J Am Geriatr Soc 1968;16(5):622–6.
7. Huntley AL, Johnson R, Purdy S, et al. Measures of multimorbidity and morbidity burden for use in primary care and community settings: a systematic review and guide. Ann Fam Med 2012;10(2):134–41.
8. Miller MD, Paradis CF, Houck PR, et al. Rating chronic medical illness burden in geropsychiatric practice and research: application of the Cumulative Illness Rating Scale. Psychiatry Res 1992;41(3):237–48.
9. Wei MY, Kabeto MU, Langa KM, et al. Multimorbidity and physical and cognitive function: performance of a new multimorbidity-weighted index. J Gerontol A Biol Sci Med Sci 2017;73(2):225–32.
10. Wei MY, Mukamal KJ. Multimorbidity, mortality, and long-term physical functioning in 3 prospective cohorts of community-dwelling adults. Am J Epidemiol 2018;187(1):103–12.
11. Sei Lee AS, Widera E. Multimorbidity-weighted index. Available at: https://eprognosis.ucsf.edu/mwi.php. Accessed.
12. Violan C, Foguet-Boreu Q, Flores-Mateo G, et al. Prevalence, determinants and patterns of multimorbidity in primary care: a systematic review of observational studies. PLoS One 2014;9(7):e102149.
13. WHO. World health statistics 2018: monitoring health for the SDGs, sustainable development goals 2018.
14. Nguyen H, Manolova G, Daskalopoulou C, et al. Prevalence of multimorbidity in community settings: a systematic review and meta-analysis of observational studies. J Comorb 2019;9. 2235042X19870934.
15. van Oostrom SH, Gijsen R, Stirbu I, et al. Time Trends in prevalence of chronic diseases and multimorbidity not only due to aging: data from general practices and health surveys. PLoS One 2016;11(8):e0160264.
16. Ward BW, Schiller JS. Prevalence of multiple chronic conditions among US adults: estimates from the National Health Interview Survey, 2010. Prev Chronic Dis 2013;10:E65.

17. Agborsangaya CB, Lau D, Lahtinen M, et al. Multimorbidity prevalence and patterns across socioeconomic determinants: a cross-sectional survey. BMC Public Health 2012;12(1):201.

18. Barnett K, Mercer SW, Norbury M, et al. Epidemiology of multimorbidity and implications for health care, research, and medical education: a cross-sectional study. Lancet 2012;380(9836):37–43.

19. Dhalwani NN, Zaccardi F, O'Donovan G, et al. Association between lifestyle factors and the incidence of multimorbidity in an older English population. J Gerontol A Biol Sci Med Sci 2016;72(4):528–34.

20. Wikström K, Lindström J, Harald K, et al. Clinical and lifestyle-related risk factors for incident multimorbidity: 10-year follow-up of Finnish population-based cohorts 1982–2012. Eur J Intern Med 2015;26(3):211–6.

21. Ruel G, Shi Z, Zhen S, et al. Association between nutrition and the evolution of multimorbidity: the importance of fruits and vegetables and whole grain products. Clin Nutr 2014;33(3):513–20.

22. Fortin M, Haggerty J, Almirall J, et al. Lifestyle factors and multimorbidity: a cross sectional study. BMC Public Health 2014;14(1):686.

23. Booth FW, Laye MJ. Lack of adequate appreciation of physical exercise's complexities can pre-empt appropriate design and interpretation in scientific discovery. J Physiol 2009;587(Pt 23):5527–39.

24. Laurin D, Verreault R, Lindsay J, et al. Physical activity and risk of cognitive impairment and dementia in elderly persons. Arch Neurol 2001;58(3):498–504.

25. Podewils LJ, Guallar E, Kuller LH, et al. Physical activity, APOE genotype, and dementia risk: findings from the cardiovascular health cognition study. Am J Epidemiol 2005;161(7):639–51.

26. Bassuk SS, Manson JE. Epidemiological evidence for the role of physical activity in reducing risk of type 2 diabetes and cardiovascular disease. J Appl Physiol 2005;99(3):1193–204.

27. Hotting K, Roder B. Beneficial effects of physical exercise on neuroplasticity and cognition. Neurosci Biobehav Rev 2013;37(9 Pt B):2243–57.

28. Hudon C, Soubhi H, Fortin M. Relationship between multimorbidity and physical activity: secondary analysis from the Quebec health survey. BMC Public Health 2008;8(1):304.

29. Autenrieth CS, Kirchberger I, Heier M, et al. Physical activity is inversely associated with multimorbidity in elderly men: results from the KORA-Age Augsburg Study. Prev Med 2013;57(1):17–9.

30. Kaplan MS, Newsom JT, McFarland BH, et al. Demographic and psychosocial correlates of physical activity in late life. Am J Prev Med 2001;21(4):306–12.

31. Farooqui AA. Effects of the high calorie diet on the development of chronic visceral disease. In: Farooqui AA, editor. High calorie diet and the human brain: metabolic consequences of long-term consumption. Cham (Switzerland): Springer International Publishing; 2015. p. 219–44.

32. Dekker LH, de Borst MH, Meems LMG, et al. The association of multimorbidity within cardio-metabolic disease domains with dietary patterns: a cross-sectional study in 129 369 men and women from the Lifelines cohort. PLoS One 2019;14(8):e0220368.

33. Shi Z, Ruel G, Dal Grande E, et al. Soft drink consumption and multimorbidity among adults. Clin Nutr ESPEN 2015;10(2):e71–6.

34. Fontana L, Hu FB. Optimal body weight for health and longevity: bridging basic, clinical, and population research. Aging Cell 2014;13(3):391–400.

35. Kivimäki M, Kuosma E, Ferrie JE, et al. Overweight, obesity, and risk of cardiometabolic multimorbidity: pooled analysis of individual-level data for 120 813 adults from 16 cohort studies from the USA and Europe. Lancet Public Health 2017;2(6):e277–85.

36. Rachel Lipari SVH. Smoking and mental illness among adults in the United States. Center for Behavioral Health Statistics and Quality, Substance Abuse and Mental Health Services Administration; 2017.

37. Castillo-Carniglia A, Keyes KM, Hasin DS, et al. Psychiatric comorbidities in alcohol use disorder. Lancet Psychiatry 2019;6(12):1068–80.

38. Centers for Disease Control and Prevention, National Center for Chronic Disease P, Health P, Office on S, Health. Publications and reports of the surgeon general. In: How tobacco smoke causes disease: the biology and behavioral basis for smoking-attributable disease: a report of the surgeon general. Atlanta (GA): Centers for Disease Control and Prevention (US); 2010.

39. Rehm J, Room R, Graham K, et al. The relationship of average volume of alcohol consumption and patterns of drinking to burden of disease: an overview. Addiction 2003;98(9):1209–28.

40. Griswold MG, Fullman N, Hawley C, et al. Alcohol use and burden for 195 countries and territories, 1990–2016: a systematic analysis for the Global Burden of Disease Study 2016. Lancet 2018;392(10152):1015–35.

41. Barnes PJ. Mechanisms of development of multimorbidity in the elderly. Eur Respir J 2015;45(3):790.

42. Betteridge DJ. What is oxidative stress? Metab Clin Exp 2000;49(2 Suppl 1):3–8.

43. Pizzino G, Irrera N, Cucinotta M, et al. Oxidative stress: harms and benefits for human health. Oxid Med Cell Longev 2017;2017:8416763.

44. Netea MG, Balkwill F, Chonchol M, et al. A guiding map for inflammation. Nat Immunol 2017;18(8):826–31.

45. Friedman E, Shorey C. Inflammation in multimorbidity and disability: an integrative review. Health Psychol 2019;38(9):791–801.

46. Friedman EM, Christ SL, Mroczek DK. Inflammation partially mediates the association of multimorbidity and functional limitations in a national sample of middle-aged and older adults: the MIDUS study. J Aging Health 2015;27(5):843–63.

47. Fabbri E, An Y, Zoli M, et al. Aging and the burden of multimorbidity: associations with inflammatory and anabolic hormonal biomarkers. J Gerontol A Biol Sci Med Sci 2015;70(1):63–70.

48. Brinkley TE, Leng X, Miller ME, et al. Chronic inflammation is associated with low physical function in older adults across multiple comorbidities. J Gerontol A Biol Sci Med Sci 2009;64(4):455–61.

49. Friedman EM, Herd P. Income, education, and inflammation: differential associations in a national probability sample (The MIDUS study). Psychosom Med 2010;72(3):290–300.

50. Gruenewald TL, Cohen S, Matthews KA, et al. Association of socioeconomic status with inflammation markers in black and white men and women in the Coronary Artery Risk Development in Young Adults (CARDIA) study. Soc Sci Med 2009;69(3):451–9.

51. Sinnige J, Braspenning J, Schellevis F, et al. The prevalence of disease clusters in older adults with multiple chronic diseases–a systematic literature review. PLoS One 2013;8(11):e79641.

52. Filipčić I, Šimunović Filipčić I, Grošić V, et al. Patterns of chronic physical multimorbidity in psychiatric and general population. J Psychosom Res 2018;114:72–80.

53. Dhar AK, Barton DA. Depression and the link with cardiovascular disease. Front Psychiatry 2016;7:33.
54. Koroukian SM, Warner DF, Owusu C, et al. Multimorbidity redefined: prospective health outcomes and the cumulative effect of co-occurring conditions. Prev Chronic Dis 2015;12:E55.
55. Wei MY, Kawachi I, Okereke OI, et al. Diverse cumulative impact of chronic diseases on physical health–related quality of life: implications for a measure of multimorbidity. Am J Epidemiol 2016;184(5):357–65.
56. Hall M, Dondo TB, Yan AT, et al. Multimorbidity and survival for patients with acute myocardial infarction in England and Wales: latent class analysis of a nationwide population-based cohort. PLoS Med 2018;15(3):e1002501.
57. Seigneurin A, Delafosse P, Tretarre B, et al. Are comorbidities associated with long-term survival of lung cancer? A population-based cohort study from French cancer registries. BMC Cancer 2018;18(1):1091.
58. Chiang JI, Jani BD, Mair FS, et al. Associations between multimorbidity, all-cause mortality and glycaemia in people with type 2 diabetes: a systematic review. PLoS One 2018;13(12):e0209585.
59. Kadam UT, Croft PR. Clinical multimorbidity and physical function in older adults: a record and health status linkage study in general practice. Fam Pract 2007;24(5):412–9.
60. Fried LP, Bandeen-Roche K, Kasper JD, et al. Association of comorbidity with disability in older women: the Women's Health and Aging Study. J Clin Epidemiol 1999;52(1):27–37.
61. Fortin M, Lapointe L, Hudon C, et al. Multimorbidity and quality of life in primary care: a systematic review. Health Qual Life Outcomes 2004;2:51.
62. Rizzuto D, Melis RJF, Angleman S, et al. Effect of chronic diseases and multimorbidity on survival and functioning in elderly adults. J Am Geriatr Soc 2017;65(5):1056–60.
63. Nguyen QD, Wu C, Odden MC, et al. Multimorbidity patterns, frailty, and survival in community-dwelling older adults. J Gerontol A Biol Sci Med Sci 2018;74(8):1265–70.
64. Fried TR, Bradley EH, Towle VR, et al. Understanding the treatment preferences of seriously ill patients. N Engl J Med 2002;346(14):1061–6.
65. Loh KP, Mohile SG, Epstein RM, et al. Willingness to bear adversity and beliefs about the curability of advanced cancer in older adults. Cancer 2019;125(14):2506–13.
66. Wei MY, Kabeto MU, Galecki AT, et al. Physical functioning decline and mortality in older adults with multimorbidity: joint modeling of longitudinal and survival data. J Gerontol A Biol Sci Med Sci 2019;74(2):226–32.
67. Jindai K, Nielson CM, Vorderstrasse BA, et al. Multimorbidity and functional limitations among adults 65 or older, NHANES 2005-2012. Prev Chronic Dis 2016;13:E151.
68. Wei MY, Levine DA, Zahodne LB, et al. Multimorbidity and cognitive decline over 14 years in older Americans. J Gerontol A Biol Sci Med Sci 2019;75(6):1206–13.
69. Fabbri E, An Y, Zoli M, et al. Association between accelerated multimorbidity and age-related cognitive decline in older Baltimore longitudinal study of aging participants without dementia. J Am Geriatr Soc 2016;64(5):965–72.
70. Vassilaki M, Aakre JA, Cha RH, et al. Multimorbidity and risk of mild cognitive impairment. J Am Geriatr Soc 2015;63(9):1783–90.
71. Wei MY, Mukamal KJ. Multimorbidity and mental health-related quality of life and risk of completed suicide. J Am Geriatr Soc 2019;67(3):511–9.

72. Makovski TT, Schmitz S, Zeegers MP, et al. Multimorbidity and quality of life: systematic literature review and meta-analysis. Ageing Res Rev 2019;53:100903.

73. Read JR, Sharpe L, Modini M, et al. Multimorbidity and depression: a systematic review and meta-analysis. J Affect Disord 2017;221:36–46.

74. Patrick L, Gaskovski P, Rexroth D. Cumulative illness and neuropsychological decline in hospitalized geriatric patients. Clin Neuropsychol 2002;16(2):145–56.

75. Moen K, Ormstad H, Wang-Hansen MS, et al. Physical function of elderly patients with multimorbidity upon acute hospital admission versus 3 weeks post-discharge. Disabil Rehabil 2018;40(11):1280–7.

76. Bahler C, Huber CA, Brungger B, et al. Multimorbidity, health care utilization and costs in an elderly community-dwelling population: a claims data based observational study. BMC Health Serv Res 2015;15:23.

77. Frolich A, Ghith N, Schiotz M, et al. Multimorbidity, healthcare utilization and socioeconomic status: a register-based study in Denmark. PLoS One 2019;14(8): e0214183.

78. Koller D, Schon G, Schafer I, et al. Multimorbidity and long-term care dependency–a five-year follow-up. BMC Geriatr 2014;14:70.

79. Wang L, Si L, Cocker F, et al. A systematic review of cost-of-illness studies of multimorbidity. Appl Health Econ Health Pol 2018;16(1):15–29.

80. Cohen HJ, Lan L, Archer L, et al. Impact of age, comorbidity and symptoms on physical function in long-term breast cancer survivors (CALGB 70803). J Geriatr Oncol 2012;3(2):82–9.

81. Kimmick GG, Li X, Fleming ST, et al. Risk of cancer death by comorbidity severity and use of adjuvant chemotherapy among women with locoregional breast cancer. J Geriatr Oncol 2018;9(3):214–20.

82. Jorgensen TL, Hallas J, Friis S, et al. Comorbidity in elderly cancer patients in relation to overall and cancer-specific mortality. Br J Cancer 2012;106(7): 1353–60.

83. Buck HG, Dickson VV, Fida R, et al. Predictors of hospitalization and quality of life in heart failure: a model of comorbidity, self-efficacy and self-care. Int J Nurs Stud 2015;52(11):1714–22.

84. Quinones AR, Markwardt S, Botoseneanu A. Diabetes-multimorbidity combinations and disability among middle-aged and older adults. J Gen Intern Med 2019;34(6):944–51.

85. Arokiasamy P, Uttamacharya U, Jain K, et al. The impact of multimorbidity on adult physical and mental health in low- and middle-income countries: what does the study on global ageing and adult health (SAGE) reveal? BMC Med 2015;13:178.

86. Su P, Ding H, Zhang W, et al. The association of multimorbidity and disability in a community-based sample of elderly aged 80 or older in Shanghai, China. BMC Geriatr 2016;16(1):178.

87. Bao J, Chua KC, Prina M, et al. Multimorbidity and care dependence in older adults: a longitudinal analysis of findings from the 10/66 study. BMC Public Health 2019;19(1):585.

Preserving Cognition, Preventing Dementia

Maryjo L. Cleveland, MD

KEYWORDS

- Dementia prevention • Prevention of cognitive decline • Lifestyle interventions

KEY POINTS

- Although dementia has often been viewed as a normal, or at least expected, sequelae of aging, there is now evidence that up to 35% of cases may be prevented.
- Early life interventions center primarily on ensuring access to 12 years of education and mitigating low socioeconomic status.
- Midlife interventions include addressing hearing loss, controlling blood pressure, and preventing obesity.
- Late-life interventions include smoking cessation, ensuring significant physical activity, treating diabetes, and minimizing depression and social isolation.
- Worldwide, multidomain intervention trials are currently under way to continue to address the issue of lifestyle approaches to prevent dementia.

INTRODUCTION

The concept of Healthy Aging is simultaneously profoundly attractive and difficult to define. In general, the notion seems to suggest aging with few disabilities and/or functional decline. Rowe and Kahn[1] define "successful aging" (which may or may not be different from "healthy aging") as "the ability to maintain 3 key behaviors or characteristics:

- Low risk of disease and disease-related disability
- High mental and physical function
- Active engagement with life"

This book, published in 1998, may have been one of the first to call out the importance of mental function. Although study after study has been undertaken with the goal of improving physical function and reducing disease, cognitive impairment was left behind. The medical community, mostly, seemed to view cognitive decline as an expected outcome of simply living long enough.

Department of Geriatrics and Gerontology, Healthy Aging and Brain Wellness Program, Wake Forest Baptist Health, Sticht Center, Medical Center Boulevard, Winston-Salem, NC 27157, USA
E-mail address: mclevela@wakehealth.edu

Clin Geriatr Med 36 (2020) 585–599
https://doi.org/10.1016/j.cger.2020.06.003
0749-0690/20/© 2020 Elsevier Inc. All rights reserved.

Epidemiologic studies regarding dementia or cognitive decline seemed to bear this out. The World Health Organization estimates that 50 million people worldwide are affected with dementia and those numbers are projected to rise to 82 million in the next decade.[2] The incidence increases exponentially with aging so that in the 65-year to 69-year-old range, there are approximately 2 new cases per 1000 persons yearly, increasing to 70 cases per 1000 persons yearly in the older than 90 age group[3] **(Fig. 1)**.

In addition, although the percentages differ based on study population, most dementia is caused by Alzheimer disease (AD), accounting for upward of 70% of all cases of dementia. AD is now the sixth leading cause of death in the United States.[4]

Fortunately, evidence is beginning to accumulate that although much of the burden of dementia is fixed by genetic and yet other unknown causes, there is a percentage; perhaps, as high as 35% that is potentially modifiable. The Lancet Commission published a thought-provoking piece in 2017 that calculated, based on accumulation of trials and epidemiologic data that outlined the contributions of primarily lifestyle choices and disease burden, the relative roles of 9 factors, occurring over 3 distinct time periods[5] **(Fig. 2)**. They have been able to estimate a population attributable fraction (PAF) for each of the factors, which represents the percentage reduction in new cases over a period of time if that particular risk factor was completely eliminated.

This article explores the data that suggest that reducing individual risk factors that may contribute to cognitive loss can ultimately reduce the development of dementia and will discuss potential interventions to mitigate these risks. Given that there is, currently, no cure for AD and it is known that AD pathology begins in the brain years, perhaps decades, before it is clinically apparent, significant attention has turned to a prevention strategy.[3] Interestingly, prevention is not the only goal that would be a "win" for the public health for our society. Even a delaying of dementia by 5 years

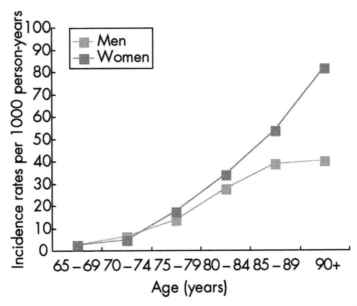

Fig. 1. Pooled incidence rates of dementia by sex. (*From* van der Flier WM, Scheltens P. Epidemiology and risk factors of dementia. J Neurol Neurosurg Psychiatry. 2005;76(suppl 5):v2-v7; with permission.)

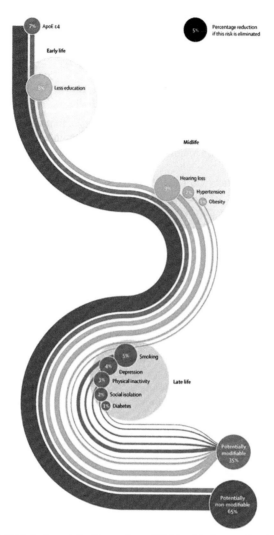

Fig. 2. Life-course model of contributions of modifiable risk factors for dementia. (Reprinted with permission from Elsevier. From Livingston G, Sommerlad A, Orgeta V, et al. Dementia prevention, intervention, and care. Lancet. 2017; 390(10113):2673-2734.)

would reduce the incidence of dementia by one-third.[6] Taken together, a delay tactic and a prevention tactic could have a profound effect on the burden of dementia worldwide.

EARLY LIFE RISK: EDUCATION

Although much work in the prevention of cognitive decline has focused on mid to late-life illnesses and lifestyle choices, there is evidence that prevention may need to begin much earlier in life. The Lancet Commission[5] estimates that the PAF for low educational level, defined as less than a high school equivalency, may account for as much as 8% of the modifiable risks for dementia.

The review by Lenehan and colleagues[7] of the relationship between education and cognitive decline suggests the following:

1. Higher levels of education predict a better performance on testing of individual cognitive domains, and yet
2. Participants with higher levels of education do not have a different trajectory of cognitive decline overall than those without (**Fig. 3**).

This dichotomy supports a "brain reserve" hypothesis: that early education provides a more robust filling of the tank. A higher degree of cognitive reserve will allow the effects of decline over time to be mitigated for longer, and for function to be higher at any point in time.

Marden and colleagues[8] also report that "education was the main contributor to cognitive reserve" versus socioeconomic status or income. Although western society has largely benefited from improved education, the challenge will be to make education available to all in less developed countries.[9]

MIDLIFE RISK FACTORS

In the Lancet Commission,[5] midlife was defined as age 45 to 65, and 3 risk factors were found to be associated with measurable PAFs: hearing loss, hypertension, and obesity.

Hearing Loss

Hearing loss (HL) is sufficiently common that patients and health care providers view it alike as "normal" or at least "benign." The prevalence of HL is nearly 50% for adults older than 60.[10] The rate continues to grow with aging, so that by age 85, the prevalence is greater than 80%. The predominant cause is loss of peripheral function; however, central auditory processing function declines with age as well. At least in part of the high prevalence, the PAF for HL is 9%.

Gurgel and colleagues[10] followed 4463 participants older than 65 who were free from dementia at baseline, in a longitudinal cohort study. Of these, 836 were found to have HL. The participants were screened regularly for cognitive change. An expert panel to determine dementia ultimately adjudicated those participants who screened

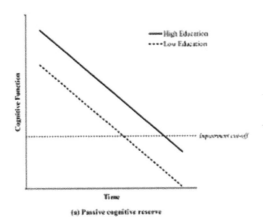

Fig. 3. The effect of education on cognitive function. (*Adapted from* Lenehan ME, Summers MJ, Saunders NL, et al. Relationship between education and age-related cognitive decline: a review of recent research. Psychogeriatrics. 2015;15(2):154–62; with permission.)

positive for cognitive impairment. Of the participants with HL, 16.3% developed dementia, compared with 12.1% of those without HL. Interestingly, HL also appeared to contribute to a more rapid acquisition of dementia, taking 10.3 years to diagnosis versus 11.9 in the normal hearing group. This outcome remained clinically significant even when controlled for gender, APOE E status, age, and baseline education. Patients with a baseline HL began the study with a lower Modified Mini-Mental State score and had a more rapid decline over the 10 years (**Fig. 4**). Participants diagnosed with mild cognitive impairment (MCI) were twice as likely to have HL as those with normal cognition. This study strongly suggests that HL is an independent risk factor for the development of cognitive impairment.

Lin and Albert[11] were also able to show that HL is associated with an accelerated rate of cognitive decline but also that the more hearing impaired the participant was, the greater their risk of developing dementia over a 10-year period (**Fig. 5**). In addition, they demonstrated that individuals with HL have accelerated rates of whole brain atrophy, particularly in the temporal region, an area important for language and semantic memory. This translated to marked impairments in tests of processing speed and executive function. They hypothesized that the relationship between HL and impaired cognition is complicated and multifactorial, with hearing loss increasing cognitive stress, changing brain structure, and causing more social isolation. These factors contribute to impaired cognitive function.

Dawes and colleagues[12] provide evidence that HL is a modifiable risk factor by showing that participants with HL who were able to obtain and use hearing aids exhibited better cognition as well as reduced social isolation and depression. Rutherford and colleagues[13] extend this to comment that hearing aids or cochlear implants improve cognitive function and reduce depressive symptoms.

As evidence accumulates that cognitive decline may be precipitated by HL, the public health imperative grows. A consistent message to older adults that HL is not normal or benign is required. Primary care physicians need to screen more

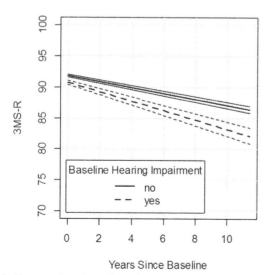

Years Since Baseline

Fig. 4. Cognitive decline as a function of HL. (*From* Gurgel RK, Ward PD, Schwartz S, et al. Relationship of hearing loss and dementia: a prospective, population-based study. Otol Neurotol. 2014;35(5):775–8; with permission.)

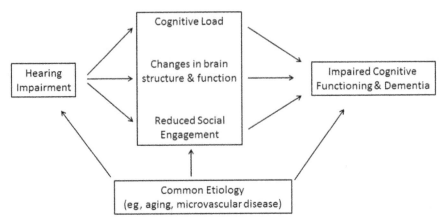

Fig. 5. Relationship between HL and dementia. (*From* Lin FR, Albert M. Hearing loss and dementia - who is listening? Aging Ment Health. 2014;18(6):671–3; with permission.)

aggressively in their practices and refer more consistently to audiologists. Finally, the cost of hearing aids, upward of $6000 each,[14] without coverage by most insurers, requires the attention of law and policy makers.

Hypertension

Hypertension has also emerged as an important midlife contributor to cognitive decline, accounting for a 2% PAF in the Lancet Commission model.[5]

Data from the Framingham offspring study showed that participants with a systolic blood pressure (BP) of greater than 140 and/or a diastolic BP of greater than 90 at midlife (mean age 55), had an elevated risk of dementia in late life with a hazard ratio of 1.57[15] (**Fig. 6**). Interestingly, for each 10-mm increment increase in BP, the risk of dementia increased, suggesting that participants with the highest BP had the highest risk of developing dementia.

Cognitive testing suggests that patients with hypertension have more impairments in executive function and processing speed than those without hypertension.[16] Hughes and Sink[17] report neuroimaging data that suggest that patients with midlife hypertension show increased total brain atrophy and smaller hippocampal brain volumes, which is highly correlated with AD. In addition, hypertension is a risk factor for small cerebral vessel disease, increasing the likelihood of vascular dementia. White matter disease burden is reduced in those with well-controlled systolic BP. Finally, autopsy data confirm that classic AD pathology (plaques and tangles) is found more frequently in those with hypertension.

Although the relationship between midlife hypertension and cognitive decline appears clear, the ability to mitigate cognitive decline with treatment of midlife BP is less so. Walker and colleagues[16] state, "Although several large placebo-controlled RCTs...have found antihypertensive agents to be protective against cognitive decline and dementia, just as many trials have failed to replicate this finding." Significant long-term study of BP intervention in mid through late life will be needed to definitively answer this question.

Obesity

The final midlife risk factor from the Lancet Commission is that of obesity, with a PAF of 1%.[5]

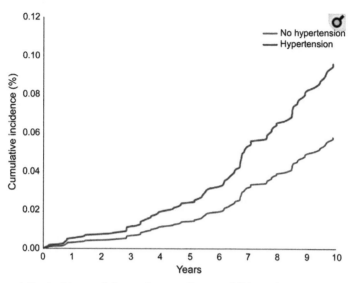

Fig. 6. Cumulative incidence of dementia according to midlife BP. (*From* McGrath ER, Beiser AS, DeCarli C, et al. Blood pressure from mid- to late life and risk of incident dementia. Neurology. 2017;89(24):2447–54; with permission.)

Obesity has become its own epidemic in the United States in recent decades. At this time, it is estimated that fully two-thirds of the US population can be categorized as overweight or obese, according to a body mass index greater than 25.[18] Obesity is related to specific impairment in cognitive domains as well as to specific neuroimaging changes.[19]

Impairment in Cognitive Domains	Neuroimaging Changes
Episodic memory	Decreased brain volume
Word list learning	Hippocampal atrophy
Working memory	Increased white matter changes

There is the suggestion that the effects of obesity on cerebral white matter ages the brain by 10 years. In addition, being obese at age 40 is estimated to increase the risk of late-life dementia by 74%. Late-life obesity, conversely, appears to be a protective factor.

The ARIC study[20] would suggest that the contribution of obesity to dementia is one of only many vascular risk factors, including smoking, diabetes, and hypertension. This observational study of more than 15,000 participants, followed from 1987 to 2011, measured vascular risk factors, demographics, and APOE E4 genotype. More than 1500 cases of dementia were diagnosed. This study was able to show that the potentially modifiable risk factors of obesity, smoking, and hypertension increased the risks for dementia, whereas hypercholesterolemia did not.

Current trends of obesity worldwide highlight need for attention to this public health issue. Estimates of dementia related to obesity would be predicted to skyrocket given the increase in obesity. However, reducing the prevalence of obesity by 20% over the next 10 years could lead to a significant reduction in dementia.[21]

Taken together, the midlife risk factors of impaired hearing, hypertension, and obesity could account for 12% of the PAF for dementia. This is not a small number.

Currently, primary care physicians focus on vascular risk factors (hypertension, smoking, diabetes) to reduce the chance of stroke and myocardial infarction. The public is well aware of these associations. It is time to add the probability that attention paid to these risk factors may also improve cognitive health outcomes.

LATE-LIFE RISK FACTORS

The Lancet Commission[5] defines late life as age older than 65 and has identified 5 areas of potentially modifiable risks: smoking, depression, physical inactivity, social isolation, and diabetes.

Smoking

The PAF related to cigarette smoking is quite high, accounting for 5%.[5] This is currently the risk with the highest late-life PAF, at least in part due to the high prevalence of smoking worldwide. Durazzo and colleagues[22] published a review of the epidemiologic evidence for smoking as a risk factor for dementia, showing changes in specific cognitive domains (processing speed, executive function, learning, and memory) in current smokers as well as changes in MRI of increased rate of global brain atrophy. Overall, smokers have a 1.7 times greater risk for AD with the risk rising with a greater "dose" of exposure.

This finding was supported by a meta-analysis by Zhong and colleagues[23] that reviewed nearly 1 million individuals, documenting nearly 15,000 cases of dementia in 37 studies (**Fig. 7**). Their primary conclusion was that current smokers have an increased risk of dementia (Relative risk 1.3) compared with never smokers. There was also evidence of a dose response, in that participants who smoked the most, had a greater incidence of dementia.

Various potential effects of cigarette smoking on the brain have been hypothesized, including increased oxidative stress, an amyloidogenic and tau pathway causing AD pathology, as well as interactions with other vascular risk factors, such as hypertension, diabetes, and obesity that predispose to VaD.

Pertinent to healthy aging, both Durazzo and colleagues[22] and Zhong and colleagues[23] conclude that former smokers did not show a similar increased risk, suggesting that smoking cessation may be a valuable intervention in the prevention of dementia.

Depression and Social Isolation

Although the Lancet Commission[5] assigns a PAF of 4 to depression and 2 to social isolation, it is difficult to tease these risk factors apart. Most studies have looked at these psychosocial risk factors as one, and they are considered so here.[24] There is considerable controversy regarding whether or not depression and social isolation are risk factors for the development of dementia, or prodromal symptoms of dementia, or actually represent a final common pathway of brain decline.

Donovan and colleagues[24] recently published data that suggest that loneliness and depression are risk factors for late-life cognitive decline. In the Health and Retirement Survey data from 1998 to 2010, participants were screened with the Center for Epidemiologic Studies Depression Scale , an 8-item depression screen with 1 question on loneliness. Cognitive testing was performed using the Telephone Interview for Cognitive Status (TICS) 10 word recall or proxy reporting. Controlling for sociodemographic differences, greater baseline loneliness predicted a 20% higher incidence of cognitive decline. In addition, the depressed groups were also associated with worsening

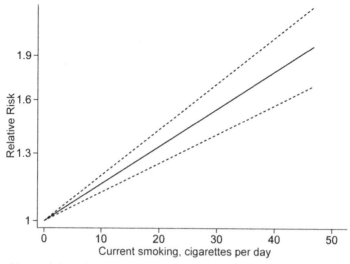

Fig. 7. Smoking and the Relative risk of dementia. (*From* Zhong G, Wang Y, Zhang Y, Guo JJ, Zhao Y. Smoking is associated with an increased risk of dementia: a meta-analysis of prospective cohort studies with investigation of potential effect modifiers. PLoS One. 2015;10(3):e0118333.)

cognition. This finding was unidirectional; low cognitive ability did not predict loneliness.

On the other hand, Singh-Manoux and colleagues[25] examined data from the Whitehall study, examining a 28-year longitudinal participant population that underwent depression screenings every 5 years. Participants were identified as having midlife versus late-life depression. Dementia was determined by survey of the electronic health record for International Classification of Diseases codes for dementia as well as by cognitive testing. They were able to show that the presence of depression early in the study (midlife) did not correlate with a higher risk for dementia, whereas those who developed late-life depression did. Depressive symptoms increased significantly in the 12 years leading up to a dementia diagnosis. These results led the investigators to dismiss the causal hypothesis and state, "these findings are consistent with the hypothesis that depressive symptoms are a prodromal feature of dementia or that the 2 share common causes."[25]

Clearly, there are factors common to both depression and dementia including poor memory, impaired sleep and changes in social function. Work needs to be done to continue to assess causality versus correlation for loneliness/depression with dementia. Regardless, evaluation and treatment of affective symptoms remain important for global well-being and may ultimately reduce the incidence of dementia.

Physical Activity

Among the most promising lifestyle interventions for the prevention of cognitive decline is exercise, with the Lancet Commission[5] assigning a PAF of 3%. This intervention is particularly attractive because of documented direct results of exercise on the brain as well as general improvements in cardiovascular function. Studies have suggested that exercise reduces cortisol, improves blood flow to the brain, maintains neural connectivity, improves brain volume (including the hippocampus), and in mouse models reduces amyloid deposition.[26] In addition, it is well-accepted that exercise improves other cardiovascular risk factors,[27] including lowering BP, lipids, and weight, all of which may contribute to AD or VaD. Unfortunately, evidence to support a relationship between inactivity and cognitive decline remains controversial.

Two recent meta-analyses have assessed the impact of physical activity on cognitive function. The first,[28] published in 2010, reviewed 15 studies representing more than 33,000 participants over 1 to 12 years and were able to show that those who engaged in a high level of physical activity had a 38% reduction in the risk of developing cognitive decline, with even low to moderate exercise resulting in benefit. Similarly, in 2017, another meta-analysis[29] reviewed more than 100,000 participants over 1 to 28 years' follow-up in 45 studies. The conclusion was also that moderate and high-intensity exercise successfully reduced the risk for developing cognitive impairment by 20%.

However, the Life Study[26] suggested the opposite. In this well-designed randomized controlled trial (RCT) of more than 1600 participants over 2 years, the investigators were unable to show any impact of moderate-intensity physical activity on global cognition or specific cognitive domains, except in those older than 80 years and those with lower baseline physical performance.

At this time, the overall conclusion remains that although RCTs have not been able to show that exercise prevents cognitive decline, there still appears to be a consistent observation that an increased "dose" of exercise is associated with a lower incidence of dementia and MCI. This remains an active area of research.[5]

Diabetes

The final risk factor discussed by the Lancet Commission[5] is related to diabetes, the presence of which appears to confer a 1% PAF.

Two recent meta-analyses support this claim. The first of these[30] reviewed 28 studies that represented data from more than 2 million individuals followed for 2 to 35 years that included 100,000 incident cases of dementia. The studies included were from Asia, Europe, and the Americas, providing a worldwide snapshot into this issue. Their findings suggested that diabetes mellitus (DM) was significantly associated with a 60% increase in dementia. Zhang and colleagues[31] performed a similar meta-analysis that pooled 17 studies representing nearly 2 million participants. Those with type 2 DM showed a significant increase in the development of AD with a relative risk of 1.53.

Data from the Gingko Evaluation of Memory Study[32] was reviewed to look at specific areas of cognitive decline in participants with and without type 2 DM. This database consisted of 3000 participants with approximately 9% having DM. Over a period of 6 years, they underwent repeated detailed cognitive testing. Global cognition declined over the course of the study; most of which was explained by the decline in executive function. The diabetic individuals in the group performed worse at baseline and actually declined more rapidly over the course of the study (**Fig. 8**).

Many mechanisms for DM causing impaired cognition have been proposed:

- Direct effects of elevated blood sugar in the brain
- Chronic hyperinsulinemia, which may increase B-amyloid
- Insulin resistance and its effects on hypertension and small vessel disease

Finally, there are data[33] that suggest that patients with amnestic MCI and DM have an increased risk of progressing to AD than those without diabetes. Most interestingly from a healthy aging point of view, those who had good control of their DM had less incidence of conversion to dementia. These data strongly suggest that DM is a modifiable risk factor. With the growing epidemic of DM, aggressive management through diet, exercise, and medication may be a rich area for dementia prevention.

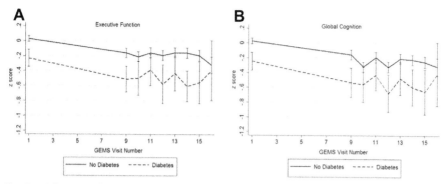

Fig. 8. Diabetes and (*A*) executive function and (*B*) global cognition. (*From* Palta P, Carlson MC, Crum RM, et al. Diabetes and cognitive decline in older adults: the ginkgo evaluation of memory study. J Gerontol A Biol Sci Med Sci. 2017;73(1):123–30; with permission.)

SUMMARY OF LANCET COMMISSION

As reviewed, the 9 potentially modifiable risk factors for dementia listed in Table 1 provide a public health platform on which an approach to reducing the incidence of dementia by 35% may be created[5] (**Table 1**).

Table 1					
Potentially modifiable factors for dementia					
Risks	**Relative Risk for Dementia (95% CI)**	**Prevalence, %**	**Communality, %**	**PAF, %**	**Weighted PAF,[a] %**
Early life (age = 18 y)					
Less education (none or primary school only)	1.6 (1.26–2.01)	40.0	64.6	19.1	7.5
Midlife (age 45–65 y)					
Hypertension	1.6 (1.16–2.24)	8.9	57.3	5.1	2.0
Obesity	1.6(1.34–1.92)	3.4	60.4	2.0	0.8
Hearing loss	1.9(1.38–2.73)	31.796	46.1	23.0	9.1
Later life (age >65 y)					
Smoking	1.6(1.15–2.20)	27.4	51 1	13 9	5.5
Depression	1.9(1.55–2.33)	13 2	58.6	10.1	4.0
Physical inactivity	1.4(1.16–1.07)	17.7	26.6	6.5	2.6
Social Isolation	1.6(1.32–1.85)	11.0	45.9	5.9	2.3
Diabetes	1.5 (1.33–1.79)	6.4	70.3	3.2	1.2

Data are relative risk (95% CI) or %. Total weighted PAF adjusted for communality = 35.0%.
Abbreviation: PAF, population attributable fraction.
[a] Weighted PAF is the relative contribution of each risk factor to the overall PAF when adjusted for communality.
Reprinted with permission from Elsevier. From Livingston G, Sommerlad A, Orgeta V, et al. Dementia prevention, intervention, and care. Lancet. 2017; 390(10113):2673-2734.

OTHERS

Data are currently unclear or contradictory for currently other potential modifiable risk factors including head trauma,[34] inadequate sleep,[35] vision loss,[36] and exposure to air pollutants,[37] among others. Ongoing research is needed to continue to evolve the model of cognitive preservation through risk factor modification.

Since the publication of the Lancet Commission, the results of the Sprint Mind data[38] were made available. The parent SPRINT study was an RCT that focused on intensive versus usual care for BP control in participants older than 50. This study was stopped early because of the positive effects on the cardiovascular endpoints, but was extended to evaluate cognitive outcomes. The SPRINT team was able to show a reduction in the incidence of MCI and a composite of MCI and dementia by 19%, although the data for dementia prevention did not reach statistical significance. SPRINT has received funding for an additional 2 years of cognitive data to help with longer-term follow-up. Therefore, hypertension appears to be a modifiable risk factor at midlife and late life.

An exciting trial conducted in Finland from 2009 to 2011, published in 2015,[39] was based on the concept of potential multidomain modifiable risk factors.

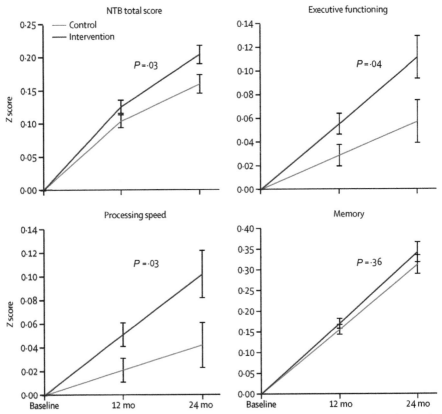

Fig. 9. Multidomain intervention on cognitive function. (*From* Ngandu T, Lehtisalo J, Solomon A, et al. A 2-year multidomain intervention of diet, exercise, cognitive training, and vascular risk monitoring versus control to prevent cognitive decline in at-risk elderly people (FINGER): a randomized controlled trial. Lancet. 2015;385(9984):2255–63; with permission.)

More than 2500 dementia-free individuals were enrolled who were at high risk for dementia based on age and presence of cardiovascular risk factors. The intervention group received intensive dietary advice, a physical activity prescription, and cognitive and social stimulation. Medical comorbidities (DM, hypertension) were managed. The control group received regular health advice. Over the 2-year study, the intervention group showed 19% less cognitive decline than the control group (**Fig. 9**).

This exciting and arguably, healthy aging approach to the prevention of cognitive decline has spawned a worldwide fingers movement, with countries all over the world participating in similar trials, including the US Pointer study, to attempt to replicate these findings.[40]

SUMMARY

Although a large percentage of patients who will develop cognitive decline will do so because of an APOE4 gene or some other yet undetermined cause, current data would suggest that approximately a third of dementia cases might be prevented by healthy living approaches.

Ensuring that everyone has access to a high-quality education for at least 12 years; screening for and providing treatment for HL; aggressively treating cardiovascular risk factors such as hypertension, DM, smoking, obesity, and low physical activity; and attending to psychosocial issues such as depression and social isolation will go a long way to mitigate the scourge of dementia and cognitive impairment.

DISCLOSURE

The author has nothing to disclose.

REFERENCES

1. Rowe JW, Kahn RL. Successful aging. Aging (Milano) 1998;10(2):142–4.
2. Hussenoeder FS, Riedel-Heller SG. Primary prevention of dementia: from modifiable risk factors to a public brain health agenda? Soc Psychiatry Psychiatr Epidemiol 2018;53(12):1289–301.
3. van der Flier WM, Scheltens P. Epidemiology and risk factors of dementia. J Neurol Neurosurg Psychiatry 2005;76(suppl 5):v2–7.
4. Alzheimer's Organization. Facts and figures. 2019. Available at: https://www.alz.org/alzheimers-dementia/facts-figures. Accessed November 1, 2019.
5. Livingston G, Sommerlad A, Orgeta V, et al. Dementia prevention, intervention, and care. Lancet 2017;390(10113):2673–734.
6. Alzheimer's Research UK. Treatment to delay dementia by five years would reduce cases by 33%. 2019. Available at: https://www.alzheimersresearchuk.org/treatment-to-delay-dementia-by-five-years-would-reduce-cases-by-33/. Accessed November 1, 2019.
7. Lenehan ME, Summers MJ, Saunders NL, et al. Relationship between education and age-related cognitive decline: a review of recent research. Psychogeriatrics 2015;15(2):154–62.
8. Marden JR, Tchetgen Tchetgen EJ, Kawachi I, et al. Contribution of socioeconomic status at 3 life-course periods to late-life memory function and decline: early and late predictors of dementia risk. Am J Epidemiol 2017;186(7):805–14.
9. Larson EB. Prospects for delaying the rising tide of worldwide, late-life dementias. Int Psychogeriatr 2010;22(8):1196–202.

10. Gurgel RK, Ward PD, Schwartz S, et al. Relationship of hearing loss and dementia: a prospective, population-based study. Otol Neurotol 2014;35(5):775–81.

11. Lin FR, Albert M. Hearing loss and dementia - who is listening? Aging Ment Health 2014;18(6):671–3.

12. Dawes P, Emsley R, Cruickshanks KJ, et al. Hearing loss and cognition: the role of hearing AIDS, social isolation and depression. PLoS One 2015;10(3):e0119616.

13. Rutherford BR, Brewster K, Golub JS, et al. Sensation and psychiatry: linking age-related hearing loss to late-life depression and cognitive decline. Am J Psychiatry 2018;175(3):215–24.

14. Healthy hearing. Hearing aid prices. 2019. Available at: https://www.healthyhearing.com/help/hearing-aids/prices. Accessed November 1, 2019.

15. McGrath ER, Beiser AS, DeCarli C, et al. Blood pressure from mid- to late life and risk of incident dementia. Neurology 2017;89(24):2447–54.

16. Walker KA, Power MC, Gottesman RF. Defining the relationship between hypertension, cognitive decline, and dementia: a review. Curr Hypertens Rep 2017; 19(3):24.

17. Hughes TM, Sink KM. Hypertension and its role in cognitive function: current evidence and challenges for the future. Am J Hypertens 2016;29(2):149–57.

18. Luchsinger JA, Gustafson DR. Adiposity and Alzheimer's disease. Curr Opin Clin Nutr Metab Care 2009;12(1):15–21.

19. Dye L, Boyle NB, Champ C, et al. The relationship between obesity and cognitive health and decline. Proc Nutr Soc 2017;76(4):443–54.

20. Gottesman RF, Albert MS, Alonso A, et al. Associations between midlife vascular risk factors and 25-year incident dementia in the atherosclerosis risk in communities (ARIC) cohort. JAMA Neurol 2017;74(10):1246–54.

21. Pedditzi E, Peters R, Beckett N. The risk of overweight/obesity in mid-life and late life for the development of dementia: a systematic review and meta-analysis of longitudinal studies. Age Ageing 2016;45(1):14–21.

22. Durazzo TC, Mattsson N, Weiner MW. Alzheimer's disease neuroimaging I. Smoking and increased Alzheimer's disease risk: a review of potential mechanisms. Alzheimers Dement 2014;10(3 Suppl):S122–45.

23. Zhong G, Wang Y, Zhang Y, et al. Smoking is associated with an increased risk of dementia: a meta-analysis of prospective cohort studies with investigation of potential effect modifiers. PLoS One 2015;10(3):e0118333.

24. Donovan NJ, Wu Q, Rentz DM, et al. Loneliness, depression and cognitive function in older U.S. adults. Int J Geriatr Psychiatry 2017;32(5):564–73.

25. Singh-Manoux A, Dugravot A, Fournier A, et al. Trajectories of depressive symptoms before diagnosis of dementia: a 28-year follow-up study. JAMA Psychiatry 2017;74(7):712–8.

26. Sink KM, Espeland MA, Castro CM, et al. Effect of a 24-month physical activity intervention vs health education on cognitive outcomes in sedentary older adults: the LIFE randomized trial. JAMA 2015;314(8):781–90.

27. Hamer M, Chida Y. Physical activity and risk of neurodegenerative disease: a systematic review of prospective evidence. Psychol Med 2009;39(1):3–11.

28. Sofi F, Valecchi D, Bacci D, et al. Physical activity and risk of cognitive decline: a meta-analysis of prospective studies. J Intern Med 2011;269(1):107–17.

29. Guure CB, Ibrahim NA, Adam MB, et al. Impact of physical activity on cognitive decline, dementia, and its subtypes: meta-analysis of prospective studies. Biomed Res Int 2017;2017:9016924.

30. Chatterjee S, Peters SA, Woodward M, et al. Type 2 diabetes as a risk factor for dementia in women compared with men: a pooled analysis of 2.3 million people

comprising more than 100,000 cases of dementia. Diabetes Care 2016;39(2): 300–7.

31. Zhang J, Chen C, Hua S, et al. An updated meta-analysis of cohort studies: diabetes and risk of Alzheimer's disease. Diabetes Res Clin Pract 2017;124:41–7.

32. Palta P, Carlson MC, Crum RM, et al. Diabetes and cognitive decline in older adults: the ginkgo evaluation of memory study. J Gerontol A Biol Sci Med Sci 2017;73(1):123–30.

33. Cooper C, Sommerlad A, Lyketsos CG, et al. Modifiable predictors of dementia in mild cognitive impairment: a systematic review and meta-analysis. Am J Psychiatry 2015;172(4):323–34.

34. Fann JR, Ribe AR, Pedersen HS, et al. Long-term risk of dementia among people with traumatic brain injury in Denmark: a population-based observational cohort study. Lancet Psychiatry 2018;5(5):424–31.

35. Spira AP, Chen-Edinboro LP, Wu MN, et al. Impact of sleep on the risk of cognitive decline and dementia. Curr Opin Psychiatry 2014;27(6):478–83.

36. Rogers MA, Langa KM. Untreated poor vision: a contributing factor to late-life dementia. Am J Epidemiol 2010;171(6):728–35.

37. Calderon-Garciduenas L, Villarreal-Rios R. Living close to heavy traffic roads, air pollution, and dementia. Lancet 2017;389(10070):675–7.

38. SPRINT MIND Investigators for the SPRINT Research Group, Williamson JD, Pajewski NM, et al. Effect of intensive vs standard blood pressure control on probable dementia: a randomized clinical trial. JAMA 2019;321(6):553–61.

39. Ngandu T, Lehtisalo J, Solomon A, et al. A 2 year multidomain intervention of diet, exercise, cognitive training, and vascular risk monitoring versus control to prevent cognitive decline in at-risk elderly people (FINGER): a randomised controlled trial. Lancet 2015;385(9984):2255–63.

40. Alzheimer's Organization. A global collaboration for future generations. 2019. Available at: https://www.alz.org/wwfingers/overview.asp. Accessed November 1, 2019.

Preserving Engagement, Nurturing Resilience

Halina Kusz, MD[a,*], Ali Ahmad, MD[b]

KEYWORDS

- Healthy aging • Resilience • Engagement • Older adults

KEY POINTS

- Healthy aging is a lifetime process that promotes an opportunity for higher quality of life in later years. Although minimizing chronic disease is important, there are many other valuable aspects of healthy aging seen by older people as more important.
- Engagement in life, active participation in family and social activities are the most important aspects of healthy aging from a layperson's perspective.
- Resilience is the ability to fully recover from stressful life events. It is perceived by older adults as an important aspect of healthy aging.
- Resilience increases with age and higher level of resilience is seen with more advanced age.
- Understanding the importance of nonbiomedical aspects of healthy aging will encourage practitioners, researchers, and policy makers to create new strategies, opportunities, and resources for healthy aging.

INTRODUCTION

The worldwide human life expectancy continues to increase. In 2018, adults reaching the age of 65 in the United States were expected to live an additional 19.5 years on average.[1] This has paved the path toward several theories and research-driven concepts in aging, such as successful, productive, and healthy aging. The World Health Organization incorporates these concepts under the term of "active aging."[2] The commonly cited Rowe and Kahn's[3] bio-medical concept of successful aging focuses on physiologic aspects of health. In this model, high level of function, absence or low risk of disease, active participation in life, and extended productive years are major determinants of successful aging.[3] In accordance with Rowe and Kahn's[3] view of

[a] Department of Medicine, Internal Medicine Residency Program, College of Human Medicine, Michigan State University, McLaren Flint, 401 South Ballenger Highway, Flint, MI 48532, USA;
[b] Geriatric Medicine, Mayo Clinic College of Medicine & Science, 200 First Street Southwest, Rochester, MN 55905, USA
* Corresponding author.
E-mail address: halina.kusz@mclaren.org

Clin Geriatr Med 36 (2020) 601–612
https://doi.org/10.1016/j.cger.2020.06.004
0749-0690/20/© 2020 Elsevier Inc. All rights reserved.

geriatric.theclinics.com

successful aging, only 11.9% of older adults in the United States demonstrate successful aging.[4]

In fact, usual aging is associated with comorbidities and a decline in cognitive and physical function. Approximately 90% of older Americans live with at least 1 chronic disease and 75% have 2 or more chronic conditions.[5] Approximately 49.8% of noninstitutionalized Americans, older than 75 years, live with 1 or more disabilities. Among them, the ambulatory disability has the highest prevalence of 32.6%.[6]

A systematic review and meta-ethnography of layperson perspectives on successful aging conducted by Cosco and colleagues[7] revealed that laypersons more commonly identified psychosocial aspects of successful aging as opposed to physiologic aspects. For example, they commonly identified social engagement and personal resources as integral components of successful aging, rather than health and longevity.[7] In a study by Carver and Buchanan,[8] several other psychological components of successful aging are highlighted, such as "engagement, resilience, optimism and/or positive attitude, spirituality and/or religiosity, self-efficacy and/or self-esteem, and gero-transcendence." This article focuses on the role, health outcomes, and practical implications of 2 major domains of healthy aging: engagement and resilience.

ENGAGEMENT

Humans have a natural desire to stay connected with people and remain actively involved in life. The sense of social connection and engagement promotes our well-being. In contrast, loneliness and social isolation negatively affect physical health, mental health, and life expectancy.[9–13] In 2018, approximately 28% of community-dwelling adults older than 65 years in the United States lived alone. This number tends to increase with advanced age.[1] Living alone, poor health, and motor impairment, are major predictors of loneliness.[14] Factors that prevent loneliness include good social support, engagement in social life, meaningful daily interactions, family life, friendships and good relationships, and overall good health. The loneliness among adults in the United States decreases with age.[15]

A literature review of articles defining attributes for social engagement include continuing to work, caring for others, and engaging in social activities. Social engagement in any meaningful life activity may benefit the health and well-being of older adults. Such engagement may be multifaceted, productive or nonproductive, and either paid or unpaid. Personal engagement and participation in family life, social networking, and social engagement represent different forms of engagement for older adults.

Personal and Family Engagement

Research reveals the health benefits of lifetime learning, engagement in creative activities, involvement in activities of daily living (ADL), and exercise and physical activities.[16,17] Family engagement becomes even more important as individuals age because needs for caregiving increase and social ties in other domains such as workplace decrease. Support from family members may promote well-being and self-esteem. Family members may provide both information and encouragement for older adults to behave in healthier ways and to better use health services. However, according to a recent study, lonely older adults are not a burden on health and social care services.[18]

Marriage

Marriage is recognized as an important promoter of health. The health benefits of marriage have been well studied by social scientists. In general, married people have better psychological well-being and are less likely to suffer mobility limitations and chronic conditions, such as diabetes, cardiovascular disease, or cancer.[19] Married people have a lower risk of mortality compared with never married, divorced, and separated people.[20]

The 2018 Profile of Older American data revealed that 70% of older American men as compared with 46% of older American women were married. Only 15% of older adults were divorced and separated. However, this percentage has increased since 1980.[1]

Caregiving and Multigenerational Living

Older adults often live together with their families and provide care to younger family members. This provides a beneficial service for the grandchildren and their parents, and simultaneously benefits the grandparents. However, some studies have found higher rate of depressive symptoms among custodial and co-parenting grandparents than among nonresidential grandparents and other noncaregivers.[21] This finding has not been reproduced in other studies.[22]

Social Relationships

Social relationships and social networking are based on interpersonal relationships with friends, neighbors, colleagues, and workplace or church members. It is an example of the informal social activity that benefits the physical and mental health of older adults. Positive social interactions decrease feelings of social isolation, and its negative impact on health[23,24] Positive relationships with family and close friends lowers the risk of depression, dementia, and mortality.[25]

Social Engagement

The aim of social engagement is to give to others. It may be informal (individual) or formal (within a group or organization) involvement. Social engagement may lead to deeper public and also political engagement. The most studied are the benefits of volunteering to both the volunteers and community.

Volunteerism

Volunteers serve the community and society beyond close family, friends, and social networking. They are engaged in social and formal activities including unpaid group activities that address community or society concerns. Several recent studies have confirmed positive associations between older people's health, well-being, quality of life, and volunteering. Volunteering buffers stress, decreases cardiovascular risks, and increases life span.[26–28] Volunteering reduces loneliness among those recently widowed,[29] and is associated with reduced risk for disabilities.[30] There is growing evidence that suggests volunteering may protect against cognitive decline.[31,32]

The positive effects of volunteering on the well-being of older adults may be seen in volunteering as little as 2 hours a week, which totals to approximately 100 hours per year.[33] One in 4 American adults are volunteers. Older adults commit more hours to volunteering than younger adults. In 2015, the age groups with the highest median hours among volunteers were ages 65 to 74 (88 hours) and those 75 and older (100 hours).[34]

RESILIENCE
What Is Resilience in Aging?

The process of aging requires the ability and endurance to face life challenges that we experience as we age. Therefore, resilience plays a crucial role in aging and takes a central place in the psychological concept of successful aging. Resiliency in aging is defined as *the ability to recover after a major stress or negative life event*. It describes a positive adaptation to the process of aging itself. It also includes adaptation to losses and adversities in later life. In the presence of challenging circumstances, resilient people recover with strength and become positively reintegrated.[35] Some philosophers and researchers view resilience as "a phenomenon," or *"a personal characteristic or trait of character."* Others see resilience as a dynamic, lifelong process that is nurtured as life goes on.[36]

Individuals who are in better physical and mental health and are socially engaged demonstrate high resilience despite stress and adversity. High resilience in later life has been also associated with improved lifestyle behaviors and better self-perception of successful aging, optimal health outcomes, and reduced depression and reduced mortality risk.[37,38] Although it is often perceived that resilience decreases with age, researchers have discovered otherwise. In fact, resilience does not decline with age, and a higher level of resilience is seen with more advanced age.[39] Personal resources, history of effective coping, and high level of social support promote resilience.

Resiliency can be assessed in older adults through resiliency measurement scales. The scales with the best psychometric ratings are shown in **Table 1**.[40–43]

There are many aspects of resiliency, and research on resilience in older adults emphasizes 2 major aspects: physiologic aspect of stress and psychological aspect of coping.[44]

Coping with Stress in Aging

Individuals are faced with challenging life circumstances; however, their responses are variable. Through adaptive capability, individuals learn how to overcome stressful events. However, intense or prolonged stress negatively influences our health and well-being. Resilient individuals tend to describe similar coping mechanisms when faced with very high levels of stress. Several strategies to cope with stress have been identified that play a crucial role in responding to difficult situations (**Box 1**).[36]

Building Cognitive, Physical, and Psychological Resilience

As we age, our cognitive and functional capacity declines. However, the rate of decline is largely related to our lifestyle.

Table 1	
Resilience scales for older adults	
Scale	**References**
Resilience Scale (RS)	Wagnild & Young,[40] 1993
Connor-Davidson Resilience Scale (CD-RISC)	Connor & Davidson,[41] 2003
Brief Resilience Scale (BRS)	Smith et al,[42] 2008

Data from Cosco TD, Kaushal A, Richards M, et al. Resilience measurement in later life: a systematic review and psychometric analysis. Health Qual Life Outcomes. 2016;14:16.

| **Box 1** |
| **Ten "Resilience Factors": mechanisms for coping with stress** |
| 1. Optimism |
| 2. Facing fear |
| 3. Moral compass, ethics, and altruism |
| 4. Religion and spirituality |
| 5. Social support |
| 6. Role models |
| 7. Training |
| 8. Brain fitness |
| 9. Cognitive and emotional flexibility |
| 10. Meaning, purpose, and growth |
| *Data from* Southwick SM, Charney DS. Resilience: the science of mastering life's greatest challenges. 2nd edition. Cambridge: Cambridge University Press; 2018. |

Diet

Healthy diet promotes overall health and well-being, and delays cognitive decline in normal aging.[45] High consumption of vegetables, fruits, and nuts is positively associated with psychological resilience.[46] Older adults recognize the importance of a healthy diet. However, there are many age-related factors that are linked to food choices. They include lifelong food preferences, retirement, bereavement, and health status, as well as environmental factors, such as transportation and social ties.[47] To promote healthier diets in older adults, we need to consider the underlying psychosocial factors that grossly influence positive effects of healthy diets on building cognitive, physical, and emotional resilience.

Physical Activity and Exercise

Both physical activity and exercise are associated with physical, cognitive, and emotional resilience, and form the essential elements of healthy aging. Aerobic exercise training is strongly associated with mental well-being. It improves memory and cognitive functions, and increases brain volume.[17,48–53] Physical activity serves as a buffer for anxiety and depression and helps improve quality of life among older adults.[54,55] As sedentary behavior is a risk factor for physical frailty,[56] the level of physical activity and exercise is inversely related to disability. Among older adults living with chronic conditions or disabilities, physical activity and exercise prevent frailty, reduce the risk of falls and fall-related injuries, and improve function and quality of life.[35]

For older adults who are physically active, at least 150 minutes to 300 minutes of exercise per week is recommended. This includes moderate-intensity aerobic physical activity and twice-weekly muscle strengthening exercises. Older adults living with chronic conditions who are unable to tolerate this recommendation should stay physically active as much as their condition allows.[57] Although physical activity and exercise can be performed individually, practicing it in a group, athletic competition, or organized charity event is more beneficial in enhancing overall resilience. It adds opportunity to build physical resilience while simultaneously engaging in social interaction.

Literature suggests that many older Americans do not achieve even the minimum amount of recommended physical activity and exercise, and approximately one-third of adults age 65 to 74 remain physically inactive.[58]

Cognitively Stimulating Activities

Lifelong learning of new information and developing new skills promote building cognitive and emotional resilience and has a positive effect on health and well-being. High cognitive performance in time of adversities positively influences the response to stress and enhances emotional resilience. Engagement in cognitively stimulating activities may prevent or slow down age-related cognitive decline and dementia.[16,59] Clinical research is emerging on brain-stimulating activities. Many brain-stimulating strategies have been developed, including online cognitive training programs for older adults.[60] Although online cognitive programs may enhance cognitive function, there is empirical evidence that shows that it may be lead to psychological distress.[61]

It has been proposed that the best way to enhance cognitive resilience is to enhance intellectual abilities according to our own capacities and interest.[36]

Psychological Well-Being

Psychological resilience refers to "the capacity to maintain, or regain, psychological well-being in the face of challenges," whereas "psychological well-being includes autonomy, environmental mastery, personal growth, positive relationships with others, and self-acceptance" (**Fig. 1**).[62] In the process of aging, 6 factors of psychological well-being overlap with psychological resilience (**Box 2**).

Psychological well-being is affected by several factors, including health, family and social relationships, social roles and activities, and factors that change with age. Evidence suggests that high level of resilience and psychological well-being may be a protective factor in health, reduce chronic medical illnesses, protect

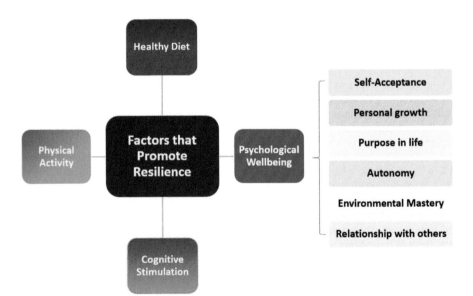

Fig. 1. The psychological well-being factors. (*Data from* Ryff CD, Keyes CLM. The structure of psychological well-being revised. J Pers Soc Psychol. 1995;69(4):719–27.)

Box 2
The psychological well-being factors that overlap with resilience in aging

1. Self-acceptance. Emphasizes the importance of positive attitude perception of self and aging.

2. Personal growth. Determines the continuation to acquire new knowledge, skills, experience.

3. Purpose in life. The finding of meaning in life and goal-oriented approach.

4. Autonomy. Preserving independence, and decision making.

5. Environmental mastery. Controlling own environment and preserving independence in activities of daily living.

6. Positive relations with others. Engaging in meaningful social relations.

Box 3
Key features of a highly resilient person[70]

A. The real patient's story:

Mrs L was a delightful and highly self-motivated woman. She suffered from many medical problems, including recurrent exacerbations of herpes simplex infection, which persisted for more than 40 years. She also suffered from diffuse degenerative joint disease, which led to many orthopedic surgeries; however, she demonstrated excellent recovery each time.

She was a widow and lived alone with her cat. She had 1 daughter who lived far away from her. She retired after 35 years of work at a local bank. She spent an additional 25 years serving as a volunteer in a community hospital. She maintained close relationships with her long-time work friends and was also closely connected to the hospital volunteer team.

She initially came to the geriatric clinic with low back pain that began following a fall. Radiographic studies confirmed the clinical diagnosis of an acute fracture of the T12 vertebral body. In addition to pain management, kyphoplasty was considered. She agreed to the therapeutic procedure; however, expressed concern that she would not be able to fulfill her duties as a volunteer.

When asked about her motivation for volunteering, she shared that, "It keeps me going. Every day, despite my pains, I get up, take care of myself and household and get ready for my work. On days I work, I take more pain medications, but working keeps me going." At her 90th birthday, she shared Henry David Thoreau's quote: "Live the life you've dreamed."

For the following 4 years, she remained independent, enjoying life, and volunteering. Unfortunately, she was diagnosed with cancer, and her health began to deteriorate. As she approached the end of life, she opted for comfort care with increased emphasis on quality of life as opposed to complex medical and surgical treatments.

Due to gradually declining physical function and increasing intractable pain, she resigned from her volunteering work. She gracefully accepted more social support that she needed and transitioned from home to the assisted living facility.

She died peacefully at the age of 96 surrounded by her family and friends. Her last wish was to die without fogging her mind with sedating medications. She asked a close friend to take care of her beloved cat.

B. Mrs L's resilience coping strategies:

- Optimism
- Acceptance
- Physical resilience
- Maintaining independence and autonomy
- Personal growth: acquiring new knowledge and skills
- Social networking and support from family and friends
- Productive engagement, engagement in volunteer work
- Finding meaning in life
- Taking full responsibility of her own life

against negative the impact of disability in later life, and promote increased survival in older adults.[63–65]

The ability to notice and regulate positive feelings predicts greater happiness, lowers depression, and improves psychological well-being.[66,67] Psychological well-being has been also associated with having a sense of purpose in life. Individuals with more role-identity absences are at risk for poorer psychological well-being. However, being a volunteer and thereby having purpose predicts positive affect.[68] In addition, as described in the previous section, psychological well-being is also mediated by physical exercise. Older adults involved in physical activity programs report significantly more adaptive emotion regulation strategies and better emotional well-being (**Box 3**).[69,70]

SUMMARY

In conclusion, aging is a lifelong process that incorporates psychosocial domains of engagement and resilience. Preserving engagement and nurturing physical, cognitive, and psychological resilience promotes positive health outcomes in later life. In recent decades, older adults have increasingly started to invest in healthy aging earlier in their lives. However, there are still many less fortunate older adults who live alone with chronic conditions, disabilities, and remain socially isolated. Every single older adult has the right to healthy aging, irrespective of race, gender, class, economic status, and location. Older adults are valuable members of our society and we need to reframe how communities view them. It therefore becomes important to acknowledge their economic and social contributions.

Research efforts from sociology, psychology, behavioral science, neuroscience, and medicine have clarified positive effects of successful aging on physical, cognitive, and emotional health. To enhance engagement and nurture resilience in older adults, we need to introduce the concept of healthy aging in our daily practice. This may include finding resources for older adults, and identifying barriers for healthy aging. Clinicians, researchers, and public policy makers should collectively develop multifaceted strategies to build healthy aging communities and societies for all older adults.

DISCLOSURE

The authors have nothing to disclose.

REFERENCES

1. Administration for community living. A profile of older Americans. 2018. Available at: https://acl.gov/aging-and-disability-in-america/data-and-research/profile-older-americans/. Accessed November 19, 2019.

2. Fernandez-Ballesteros R, Robine JM, Walker A, et al. Active aging: a global goal. Curr Gerontol Geriatr Res 2013;2013:298012.

3. Rowe JW, Kahn RL. Successful aging. Gerontologist 1997;37(4):433–40.

4. McLaughlin SJ, Connell CM, Heeringa SG, et al. Successful aging in the United States: prevalence estimates from a national sample of older adults. J Gerontol B Psychol Sci Soc Sci 2010;65B(2):216–26.

5. National Council on Aging. Fact sheet: healthy aging 2014. Available at: https://www.ncoa.org/resources/fact-sheet-healthy-aging/. Accessed November 19, 2019.

6. Erickson W, Lee C, von Schrader S. 2015 disability status report : United States. 2016. Available at: http://www.disabilitystatistics.org/StatusReports/2015-PDF/2015-StatusReportUS.pdf/. Accessed November 19, 2019.

7. Cosco TD, Prina AM, Perales J, et al. Lay perspectives of successful ageing: a systematic review and meta-ethnography. BMJ Open 2013;3(6):1–9.

8. Carver LF, Buchanan D. Successful aging: considering non-biomedical constructs. Clin Interv Aging 2016;11:1623–30.

9. Cacioppo JT, Cacioppo S. The growing problem of loneliness. Lancet 2018; 391(10119):426.

10. Cacioppo JT, Cacioppo S. Older adults reporting social isolation or loneliness show poorer cognitive function 4 years later. Evid Based Nurs 2014;17(2):59–60.

11. Holt-Lunstad J, Smith TB. Loneliness and social isolation as risk factors for CVD: implications for evidence-based patient care and scientific inquiry. Heart 2016; 102(13):987–9.

12. Holt-Lunstad J, Smith TB, Baker M, et al. Loneliness and social isolation as risk factors for mortality: a meta-analytic review. Perspect Psychol Sci 2015;10(2): 227–37.

13. Luo Y, Hawkley LC, Waite LJ, et al. Loneliness, health, and mortality in old age: a national longitudinal study. Soc Sci Med 2012;74(6):907–14.

14. Theeke LA. Predictors of loneliness in U.S. adults over age sixty-five. Arch Psychiatr Nurs 2009;23(5):387–96.

15. Bruce LD, Wu JS, Lustig SL, et al. Loneliness in the United States: a 2018 national panel survey of demographic, structural, cognitive, and behavioral characteristics. Am J Health Promot 2019;33(8):1123–33.

16. Klimova B. Learning a foreign language: a review on recent findings about its effect on the enhancement of cognitive functions among healthy older individuals. Front Hum Neurosci 2018;12:305.

17. Windle G, Hughes D, Linck P, et al. Is exercise effective in promoting mental well-being in older age? A systematic review. Aging Ment Health 2010;14(6):652–69.

18. Valtorta NK, Moore DC, Barron L, et al. Older adult's social relationships and health care utilization: a systematic review. Am J Public Health 2018;108(4): e1–10.

19. Wood RG, Goesling B, Avellar S. The effect of marriage on health: a synthesis of current research evidence. 2007. Available at: https://aspe.hhs.gov/system/files/pdf/180036/rb.pdf/. Accessed December 2, 2019.

20. Kaplan RM, Kronick RG. Marital status and longevity in the United States population. J Epidemiol Community Health 2006;60(9):760–5.

21. Musil CM, Gordon NL, Warner CB, et al. Grandmothers and caregiving to grandchildren: continuity, change, and outcomes over 24 months. Gerontologist 2011; 51(1):86–100.

22. Hughes ME, Waite LJ, LaPierre TA, et al. All in the family: the impact of caring for grandchildren on grandparents' health. J Gerontol B Psychol Sci Soc Sci 2007; 62(2):S108–19.

23. Choi H, Irwin MR, Cho HJ. Impact of social isolation on behavioral health in elderly: systematic review. World J Psychiatry 2015;5(4):432–8.

24. Cho JH, Olmstead R, Choi H, et al. Associations of objective versus subjective social isolation with sleep disturbance, depression, and fatigue in community-dwelling older adults. Aging Ment Health 2019;(9):1130–8.

25. Umberson D, Montez JK. Social relationships and health: a flashpoint for health policy. J Health Soc Behav 2010;51:S54–66.

26. Han SH, Kim K, Burr JA. Stress-buffering effects of volunteering on daily well-being: evidence from the National Study of Daily Experiences. J Gerontol B Psychol Sci Soc Sci 2019. https://doi.org/10.1093/geronb/gbz052.

27. Han SH, Tavares JL, Evans M, et al. Social activities, incident cardiovascular disease, and mortality. J Aging Health 2017;2(2):268–88.

28. Okun MA, Yeung EW, Brown S. Volunteering by older adults and risk of mortality: a meta-analysis. Psychol Aging 2013;28(2):564–77.

29. Carr DC, Kail BL, Matz-Costa C, et al. Does becoming a volunteer attenuate loneliness among recently widowed older adults? J Gerontol B Psychol Sci Soc Sci 2018;73(3):501–10.

30. Carr DC, Kail BL, Rowe JW. The relation of volunteering and subsequent changes in physical disability in older adults. J Gerontol B Psychol Sci Soc Sci 2018;73(3):511–21.

31. Guiney H, Machado L. Volunteering in the community: potential benefits for cognitive aging. J Gerontol B Psychol Sci Soc Sci 2018;73(3):399–408.

32. Proulx CM, Curl AL, Ermer AE. Longitudinal associations between formal volunteering and cognitive functioning. J Gerontol B Psychol Sci Soc Sci 2018;73(3):522–31.

33. Morrow-Howell N, Hinterlong J, Rozario A, et al. The effect of volunteering on the well-being of older adults. J Gerontol B Psychol Sci Soc Sci 2003;58B(3):S137–45.

34. Corporation for National and Community Service. 2016 new report: service unites Americans; volunteers give service worth $184billion. Available at: https://www.NationalService.gov. Accessed November 25, 2019.

35. Resnick B, Gwyther LP, Roberto KA. Conclusion: the key to successful aging. In: Resnick B, Gwyther L, Roberto K, editors. Resilience in aging. 2nd edition. Cham (Switzerland): Springer; 2018. p. 401–15.

36. Southwick SM, Charney DS. What is resilience?. In: Southwick SM, Charney DS, editors. Resilience: the science of mastering life's greatest challenges. 2nd edition. Cambridge (England): Cambridge University Press; 2018. p. 1–34.

37. Moore RC, Eyler LT, Mausbach BT, et al. Complex interplay between health and successful aging: role of perceived stress, resilience, and social support. Am J Geriatr Psychiatry 2015;23(6):622–32.

38. Jeste DV, Savla GN, Thompson WK, et al. Association between older age and more successful aging: critical role of resilience and depression. Am J Psychiatry 2013;170(2):188–96.

39. MacLeod S, Musich S, Hawkins K, et al. The impact of resilience among older adults. Geriatr Nurs 2016;3794:266–72.

40. Wagnild GM, Young HM. Development and psychometric evaluation of the resilience scale. J Nurs Meas 1993;1(2):165–78.

41. Connor KM, Davidson JR. Development of a new resilience scale: the Connor-Davidson Resilience Scale (CD-RISC). Depress Anxiety 2003;18(2):76–82.

42. Smith BW, Dalen J, Wiggins K, et al. The brief resilience scale: assessing the ability to bounce back. Int J Behav Med 2008;15(3):194–200.

43. Cosco TD, Kaushal A, Richards M, et al. Resilience measurement in later life: a systematic review and psychometric analysis. Health Qual Life Outcomes 2016;14:16.

44. Southwick SM, Bonanno GA, Masten AS, et al. Resilience definitions, theory, and challenges: interdisciplinary perspectives. Eur J Psychotraumatol 2014;5(10):1–14.

45. Klimova B, Valis M. Nutritional interventions as beneficial strategies to delay cognitive decline in healthy older individuals. Nutrients 2018;10(7):10.
46. Yin Z, Brasher MS, Kraus VB, et al. Dietary diversity was positively associated with psychological resilience among elders: a population-based study. Nutrients 2019;11(3):10.
47. Bloom I, Lawrence W, Barker M, et al. What influences diet quality in older people? A qualitative study among community-dwelling older adults from the Hertfordshire Cohort Study, UK. Public Health Nutr 2017;20(15):2685–93.
48. Colcombe SJ, Erickson KI, Scalf PE, et al. Aerobic exercise training increases brain volume in aging humans. J Gerontol A Biol Sci Med Sci 2006;61(11):1166–70.
49. Erickson KI, Voss MW, Prakash RS, et al. Exercise training increases size of hippocampus and improves memory. Proc Natl Acad Sci U S A 2011;108(7):3017–22.
50. Jackson PA, Pialoux V, Corbett D, et al. Promoting brain health through exercise and diet in older adults: a physiological perspective. J Physiol 2016;594(16):4485–98.
51. Prakash RS, Voss MW, Erickson KI, et al. Physical activity and cognitive vitality. Annu Rev Psychol 2015;66:769–97.
52. Voss MW, Heo S, Prakash RS, et al. The influence of aerobic fitness on cerebral white matter integrity and cognitive function in older adults: results of a one-year exercise intervention. Hum Brain Mapp 2013;34(11):2972–85.
53. Weinstein AM, Voss MW, Prakash RS, et al. The association between aerobic fitness and executive function is mediated by prefrontal cortex volume. Brain Behav Immun 2012;26(5):811–9.
54. Schuch FB, Stubbs B, Meyer J, et al. Physical activity protects from incident anxiety: a meta-analysis of prospective cohort studies. Depress Anxiety 2019;36(9):846–58.
55. Schuch FB, Vancampfort D, Richards J, et al. Exercise as a treatment for depression: a meta-analysis adjusting for publication bias. J Psychiatr Res 2016;77:42–51.
56. Song J, Lindquist LA, Chang RW, et al. Sedentary behavior as a risk factor for physical frailty independent of moderate activity: results from the osteoarthritis initiative. Am J Public Health 2015;105(7):1439–45.
57. Office of Disease Prevention and Health Promotion. Physical activity guidelines for Americans. 2018. Available at: https://health.gov/paguidelines/second-edition/pdf/PAG_ExecutiveSummary.pdf/. Accessed November 26, 2019.
58. Elsawy B, Higgins KE. Physical activity guidelines for older adults. Am Fam Physician 2010;81(1):55–9.
59. Qiu C, Fratiglioni L. Aging without dementia is achievable. J Alzheimers Dis 2018;62:933–42.
60. Klimova B. Use of the Internet as a prevention tool against cognitive decline in normal aging. Clin Interv Aging 2016;11:1231–7.
61. Wu AMS, Chen JH, Tong KK, et al. Prevalence and associated factors of internet gaming disorder among community dwelling adults in Macao, China. J Behav Addict 2018;7(1):62–9.
62. Ryff CD, Keyes CLM. The structure of psychological well-being revised. J Pers Soc Psychol 1995;69(4):719–27.
63. Steptoe A, Deaton A, Stone AA. Subjective wellbeing, health, and ageing. Lancet 2015;385(9968):640–8.

64. Manning LK, Carr DC, Kail BL. Do higher levels of resilience buffer the deleterious impact of chronic illness on disability in later life? Gerontologist 2016;56(3): 514–24.

65. Chida Y, Steptoe A. Positive psychological well-being and mortality: a quantitative review of prospective observational studies. Psychosom Med 2008;70(7):741–56.

66. Smith JL, Hollinger-Smith L. Savoring, resilience, and psychological well-being in older adults. Aging Ment Health 2015;19(3):192–200.

67. Smith JL, Hanni AA. Effects of a savoring intervention on resilience and well-being of older adults. J Appl Gerontol 2019;38(1):137–52.

68. Greenfield EA, Marks NF. Formal volunteering as a protective factor for older adults' psychological well-being. J Gerontol B Psychol Sci Soc Sci 2004;59(5): S258–64.

69. Delle Fave A, Bassi M, Boccaletti ES, et al. Promoting well-being in old age: the psychological benefits of two training programs of adapted physical activity. Front Psychol 2018;9:828.

70. Kusz H, Smith S, Dohrenwend A. What does volunteering mean for the patient with chronic pain? Poster presented at the 7th International Association of Gerontology and Geriatrics European Congress, Bologna, Italy, April 14-17, 2011.

Reducing Frailty to Promote Healthy Aging

Veronica C. Nwagwu, MD[a],*, Christine Cigolle, MD[b], Theodore Suh, MD, PhD[a]

KEYWORDS

- Multicomponent frailty intervention model • Functional decline • Healthy aging

KEY POINTS

- Unexplained weight loss, exhaustion, weakness, slow walking speed, and low physical activity are important red flags of frailty. Exercise, cognitive stimulation, improving sleep, nutrition, and social interaction are part of a multidomain approach to reduce frailty and promote healthy aging.
- It may be most beneficial to target pre-frail older adults with interventions listed above, to potentially mitigate progression from pre-frailty to frailty.

INTRODUCTION

Over the past century, life expectancy has significantly increased worldwide. It is projected that between 2000 and 2050, the number of people aged 60 years or older in the world will double from about 11% to 22%, an increase from approximately 605 million to 2 billion.[1] By 2050, life expectancy will likely exceed 90 years of age.[2]

The number of older adults aged older than 80 years is expected to quadruple to 395 million during the same period; this increase in life expectancy allows for older adults to develop chronic diseases, which ultimately predisposes them to disability, dependency, or frailty.[1]

The term "frailty" refers to age-related vulnerability and functional decline, which increases susceptibility to adverse health outcomes. Frailty is now considered a medical syndrome rather than a single disease entity.[3]

Frail older patients have progressive functional decline with markedly low functional reserve, and they are vulnerable to adverse outcomes in various clinical settings (including but not limited to), such as, postsurgical complications, falls, institutionalization, disability, and even death.[4] Thus, it is important to identify frail older adults with highest risk for adverse outcomes before embarking on surgical procedures, in other words, to choose safer and more appropriate treatment options.[3]

[a] Geriatric Center, University of Michigan, 4260 Plymouth Road, Ann Arbor, MI 48109, USA;
[b] Geriatric Research Education and Clinical Center (GRECC), Veterans Affairs Ann Arbor 2215 Fuller Road, Ann Arbor, MI 48105, USA
* Corresponding author.
E-mail addresses: docveronica.md@gmail.com; vnwagwu@med.umich.edu

Clin Geriatr Med 36 (2020) 613–630
https://doi.org/10.1016/j.cger.2020.06.005
0749-0690/20/© 2020 Elsevier Inc. All rights reserved.

Presurgical screening for frailty may provide a premise to develop interventions to decrease unplanned readmissions and complications after medical or surgical procedures.[5]

This article reviews the concept and definition of frailty, epidemiology, pathophysiology, frailty framework, risk factors, tools for clinical assessment, complications of frailty, and tips to reduce frailty to promote healthy aging.

DEFINITION

Several definitions of frailty have been proposed; there have been divided opinions and no consensus on whether frailty should be defined solely in terms of biomedical factors or whether psychosocial aspects should be considered in the definition.

Frailty is generally considered to be a medical syndrome with multifactorial cause and risk factors, characterized by diminished strength and endurance as well as compromised physiologic function, leading to increased vulnerability for adverse health outcomes, including early mortality.[3]

The World Health Organization (WHO) conceptually defines frailty as "a clinically recognizable state in which the ability of older people to cope with acute stressors is compromised by an increased vulnerability due to age-associated declines in physiological reserve and function across multiple organ systems."[6]

Although old age is associated with increased prevalence of frailty, old age by itself does not define or establish the diagnosis of frailty. Some older adults remain high functioning, robust, and vigorous despite advanced age; hence, poor functional status (an important aspect of frailty) is a nonstatic, dynamic process not simply explained by age.

COMPONENTS OF FRAILTY

Frailty has 3 important components: physical, psychological, and sociologic frailty; all 3 components interact in a complex way in a frail elderly patient, as shown in **Fig. 1**.

EPIDEMIOLOGY
Age

In the Cardiovascular Health Study (CHS), the overall prevalence of frailty ranges between 7% and 12% in community-dwelling adults aged 65 or older in the United States.[7] Advanced age is a significant risk factor for frailty, and a quarter of those aged 80 years and older are frail.[8]

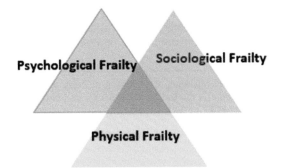

Fig. 1. Components of frailty.

Gender

The CHS study demonstrated that the prevalence of frailty was greater in women than men (8% vs 5%).[7]

Race

African Americans were more than twice as likely to be frail AS Caucasians in CHS (13% vs 6%, although prevalence of frailty among Hispanic Americans was 7.8%, similar to those of Caucasians according to data from Hispanic Established Populations for Epidemiologic Studies of the Elderly.[7]

Comorbidities

A higher prevalence of frailty is also observed with specific diseases/comorbidities, such as patients with

- Cancer (42%),[9] end-stage renal disease (37%),[10] heart failure (45%)[11]
- Alzheimer disease (32%),[12] nursing home residents (52%)[13]

Fig. 2 shows prevalence of frailty based on various comorbidities.

THE CYCLE OF LIFE

The Famous Ancient Greek "Riddle of the Sphinx" is a good reminder of the overall cycle of life as one ages.

The riddle: what has 4 legs in the morning, 2 legs at noon, and 3 legs in the evening?
The answer (by Oedipus in the Greek myth): A man (referring to human being)
A man is a baby (in the "morning of his life") and crawls on 4 feet.
A man is an adult (at the "noon/middle part of his life") and he walks on 2 feet.
When a man is old ("in the evening time of his life"), he uses a cane, walking on 3 feet.

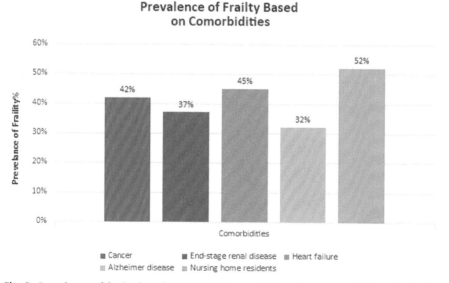

Prevalence of Frailty Based on Comorbidities

■ Cancer   ■ End-stage renal disease   ■ Heart failure
■ Alzheimer disease   ■ Nursing home residents

Fig. 2. Prevalence of frailty based on various comorbidities. (*Data from* Walston JD. Frailty. Available at: https://www.uptodate.com/contents/frailty.)

Frailty as a geriatric syndrome commonly affects older adults "in the evening phase" of their lives.

Fig. 3 shows the aging journey.

Interventions should be targeted at the prefrail stage for best results to delay further progression to full-blown frailty or to reverse the process of decline.

PROGRESSION OF FRAILTY (FRAILTY SPECTRUM)

Fried's frailty phenotype is defined by 5 criteria: exhaustion, unexplained weight loss, weakness, slowness, and low physical activity. Prefrailty meets 1 or 2 of these 5 criteria.

Fig. 4 shows the cascade of functional decline in older adults from independence, through to frailty and disability (in the absence of intervention).[14]

The frailty spectrum can be theoretically stretched further from disability to failure to thrive and finally death: *Robustness → Prefrail → Frail → Disability → Failure to Thrive → High Risk for Death/Mortality.*

PATHOPHYSIOLOGY OF FRAILTY

There is increasing evidence that dysregulation in multiple systemic pathways, including immune, endocrine, metabolic, nutrition, and energy response systems, plays an important role in developing frailty.[3] This multisystemic dysregulation seems to be driven by complex molecular changes related to aging, stress, and genetics; they are further modified by underlying disease states, leading to physiologic derangements and loss of muscle mass (sarcopenia), which ultimately manifests as clinical frailty.

- *Endocrine*: Data suggest that reduced growth hormone and insulin-like growth factor may be associated with lower strength and decreased mobility in community-dwelling older women,[15] while increased stress hormone cortisol can worsen the burden of frailty.[16,17]
- *Inflammation and the immune system*: There is evidence to support the strong correlation between frailty and biomarkers of the immune system. Stress hormones, proinflammatory cytokine, interleukin-6), and C-reactive protein can adversely impact skeletal muscle; thus, they were found elevated in community-dwelling frail older adults.[18,19]
- *Nutrition:* Studies suggest that low protein consumption may predispose to sarcopenia and frailty in older adults through complex mechanisms.[20] The concept of anabolic resistance is important to better understand the complex interaction

Best time for interventions to prevent frailty

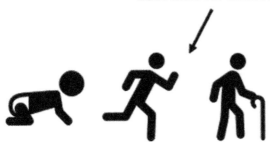

Fig. 3. Illustration of the aging process.

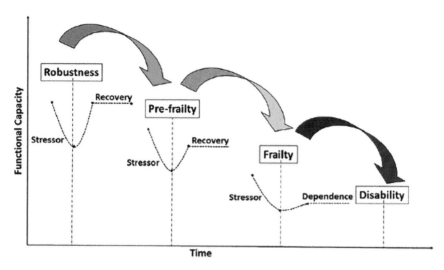

Fig. 4. Progression of Frailty (Frailty Spectrum). *From* Dent E, Morley JE, Cruz-Jentoft AJ, et al. Physical frailty: ICFSR international clinical practice guidelines for identification and management. J Nutr Health Aging. 2019;23(9):773. http://creativecommons.org/licenses/by/4.0/

between nutrition and frailty. Frail older adults tend to have reduced muscle sensitivity to circulating amino acids, leading to decreased muscle uptake of amino acids. This causes ineffective use of available proteins for muscle building.

- *Homeostenosis and Loss of Resilience:* Homeostenosis is a relevant concept in geriatrics and gerontology. The term "stenosis" is used to describe narrowing of a structure; thus, homeostenosis refers to narrowing or limitation in the body's ability to maintain homeostasis/equilibrium.[21] In a healthy young person, the body has the remarkable ability to repair itself during stress, illness, or disease. The body typically uses its physiologic and functional reserves during stress to maintain stability and restore equilibrium, as seen in **Fig. 5**.

As one gets older, the body's physiologic and functional reserves diminish progressively, thus limiting the older adults' ability to mount resistance to stress, thereby increasing their vulnerability to illness. If stress gets extreme and prolonged, the aging body uses up its functional reserve quickly, leading to *loss of resilience* and ultimately *decompensation*, thus resulting in illness, organ damage, and even *potential death*. Stressors/insult may include trauma, injury, emotional disturbance, grief following loss of loved one, loss of income, stress of surgery or medical interventions, new medication with side effects, and more.[21]

Robust people are regarded as fully resilient, and prefrail adults have compromised resilience, whereas frail older adults lack resilience and have marked vulnerability to morbidity and mortality. It is important to keep older adults mentally and medically optimized to give them the best fighting chance should they get hit by illness or acute life stressors.

THE FRAILTY FRAMEWORK

The pathogenesis of frailty as demonstrated in **Fig. 6** shows how the aging older adult when challenged with chronic illness and multiple comorbidities undergoes an array of dysregulated immune, endocrine, and metabolic changes, including increased insulin resistance, oxidative stress, low-grade inflammation, protein degradation, increased

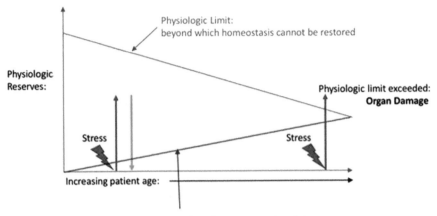

Fig. 5. Homeostenosis. (*From* Whittle J, Wischmeyer PE, Grocott MPW, et al. Surgical prehabilitation: nutrition and exercise. Anesthesiol Clin. 2018;36(4):569; with permission.

intramuscular/visceral fat deposition with paradoxic reduced protein synthesis, and diminished muscle blood flow among others. These dysregulated changes herald development of sarcopenia (noticeable loss of muscle mass). Sarcopenia seems to be an important hallmark of clinical frailty.

The frail older adult exhibits diminished physical activity, slow gait speed, poor grip strength, exhaustion, fatigue, weight loss, and heightened vulnerability to physical and psychological stressors, which negatively impact physical and cognitive function and ultimately increases adverse medical outcomes like disability, increased dependence on caregivers, institutionalization, hospitalization, and even death.

RISK FACTORS FOR FRAILTY

In addition to sarcopenia and worsening chronic illnesses, other modifiable and non-modifiable risk factors associated with increased prevalence of frailty include the following:

- Older age[22]
- Lower education level[22]
- Current smoker[22]
- Current use of postmenopausal hormone therapy[22]
- Not married[23]
- African American or Hispanic ethnicity (in a US sample)[24]
- Depression or use of antidepressants[25]
- Intellectual disability/cognitive impairment[26]

CLINICAL ASSESSMENT/SCREENING TOOLS
Why Screen for Frailty?

Identifying frail adults is a public health interest. Thus, the US Preventive Service Task Force recommends that health practitioners screen older adults for frailty using a validated instrument suitable for the specific setting or context; for individuals who screened positive for frailty, a more comprehensive clinical assessment should be performed to identify signs and underlying mechanisms of frailty (strong recommendation).[14]

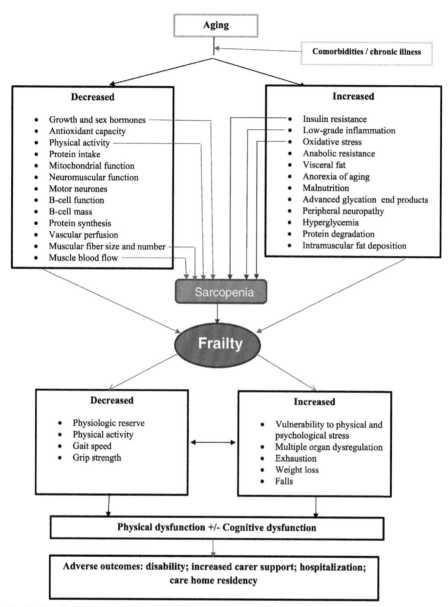

Fig. 6. The frailty framework. (*From* Sinclair AJ, Abdelhafiz AH, Rodríguez-Mañas L. Frailty and sarcopenia - newly emerging and high impact complications of diabetes. J Diabetes Complications. 2017;31(9):1467; with permission.)

Case Description

Mr Patrick is a 92-year-old retired veteran who is "shrinking." He has lost 12 kg (26 pounds) unintentionally over the past 20 months. He has become more "wobbly," and unsteady and has fallen several times. He now uses a walker for extra support. He reports "loss of strength" and notably walks *slowly*. He endorses occasional urinary retention, which has occurred intermittently for several years. This seems to be triggered by taking cold-remedy medications available over the counter.

His medical history includes a mini-stroke (transient ischemic attack), psoriatic arthritis in remission, well-controlled hypertension, atrial fibrillation, hyperlipidemia, and type 2 diabetes. He is widowed and currently lives independently with his adult daughter.

Mr Patrick visits his urologist for blood in the urine and worsening urinary retention. Physical examination reveals notably slow gait, generally reduced muscle mass, and noticeable weight loss. Urine culture is clear, and no urinary tract infection is identified. Results of a bladder scan showed a postvoid residual volume of 400 cc of urine. Cystoscopy is arranged under spinal anesthesia, and he is sent home with an indwelling Foley catheter.

During the next 3 days, Mr Patrick develops confusion and experiences repeated falls. He now needs assistance from 2 people to transfer and requires assistance with feeding and toileting. His daughter (who works full time) is no longer able to manage his care needs. He is sent to the emergency department for increased confusion, where he is diagnosed with new pneumonia and elevated cardiac enzymes because of demand-supply myocardial infarction. He also had new hyponatremia and has become more delirious.

He is admitted to the hospital for intravenous antibiotics, fluids, and management of electrolytes. Physical therapy evaluation is recommending need for eventual subacute rehabilitation after current hospital stay.[27]

This case clearly demonstrates the potential disastrous effects of frailty, a state of increased vulnerability to poor outcomes with reduced ability to recover from an acute stressor. For this frail senior, a minor medical procedure has resulted in serious adverse outcomes.[27] Ongoing advocacy to screen older adults for frailty before elective procedures/surgery helps to identify 'at risk' individuals before they get exposed to procedures that may result in adverse outcomes.

SCREENING TOOLS FOR FRAILTY

A weakness in the science of frailty is the lack of consensus in the definition and absence of a gold-standard tool for screening. For a good geriatrician, you know frailty when you see it; however, it helps to use a screening tool for a more objective assessment.

The Fried or Hopkins Frailty Phenotype

This tool was developed by Fried and colleagues[4] using the CHS cohort in 2001.

> Pros: This is the most commonly cited frailty screening tool and has been validated in the CHS.[3]
> Cons: It requires patient participation to measure gait speed and specialized equipment for grip strength measurement.

A positive screen for frailty is 3 or more out of these 5 criteria:

- Weight loss ($\geq$5% of body weight in the last year)
- Exhaustion (positive response to questions regarding effort required for activity)
- Weakness (decreased grip strength)
- Slow walking speed (gait speed) (>6–7 seconds to walk 15 feet)
- Decreased physical activity (Kcals spent per week: men expending <383 Kcals and women <270 Kcal)

"Prefrailty" is defined as 1 or 2 out of these 5 criteria; "not frail" (robust) is defined as having none.

The Deficit Accumulation or Index Approach

In contrast to the frailty phenotype, this tool, described by Rockwood and Mitnitski,[28] measures frailty based on the accumulation of illnesses, functional and cognitive declines, and social situations that are added together to calculate frailty. It requires answering 20 or more medical and functional-related questions. The higher the number of deficits, the higher the frailty score.[3]

> *Pros:* The tool does not require physical examination to assess frailty. It can be adapted to information available in the medical record.[3]
> *Cons:* It can be time consuming in a busy clinic.

The "FRAIL" Scale

The "*FRAIL*" scale is a tool that takes only minutes to perform and can be incorporated into the history-taking part. The mnemonic "FRAIL" is helpful in remembering the component questions:

- *Fatigue* ("Have you felt fatigued? Most or all of the time over the past month?")
  Yes = score 1, No = score 0
- *Resistance* ("Do you have difficulty climbing a flight of stairs?")
  Yes = score 1, No = score 0
- *Ambulation* ("Do you have difficulty walking 1 block?")
  Yes = score 1, No = score 0
- *Illnesses* ("Do you have any of these illnesses: hypertension, diabetes, cancer [other than a minor skin cancer], chronic lung disease, heart attack, congestive heart failure, angina, asthma, arthritis, stroke, and kidney disease?")
  Five or greater = score 1, fewer than 5 = score 0
- *Loss of weight* ("Have you lost more than 5% of your weight in the past year?")
  Yes = score 1, No = score 0
  Frail scale scores range from 0 to 5 (0 = best, 5 = worst)
  ○ Frail = (3–5) score, prefrail = (1 to 2) score, robust health status= (0) score.[3]

The Study of Osteoporotic Fractures Frailty Tool

The study of osteoporotic fractures frailty tool is another tool known for its ease in administering in most clinical settings. Frailty is defined by this tool as the presence of at least 2 of 3 components:

- *Weight loss of 5 percent in last year;*
- *Inability to rise from a chair 5 times without use of arms; or*
- *A "no" response to the question, "Do you feel full of energy?"*[29]

There are several other tools described in the literature for screening purposes: Clinical Frailty Scale, Edmonton Frail Scale, INTER-FRAIL, Prisma-7, Sherbrooke Postal Questionnaire, Short Physical Performance Battery, The Kihon Checklist, a self-reported comprehensive questionnaire, The Frailty Index for Elders, and many others.

Gait Speed: An Important Measure of Frailty

There are robust data to support that gait speed in older adults is an important and sensitive measure of frailty. It has been accepted as a reliable predictor of adverse clinical outcomes, and hence, gait speed is regarded as the "sixth vital sign."[30]

The International Academy on Nutrition and Aging 2009 found that among ambulatory elderly patients, a slow gait speed over a distance of 4 m was predictive of mortality (threshold of 1 m/s), and slow gait speed was further predictive of adverse medical complications, including hospitalization, disability, falls, and cognitive decline, with a threshold of 0.8 m/s.[31]

Another study reports that for every 0.1 m/s decrease in walking speed, the risk of dying or unplanned hospital or emergency room use increased by 22%, 33%, and 34%, respectively, among patients with cancer; gait speed remained an independent predictor of death in this study.[32]

COMPLICATIONS OF FRAILTY

In a study of 594 older adults, Johns Hopkins researchers have found that frailty

- Doubles the risk of surgical complications,
- Lengthens hospital stays,
- Increases the odds of moving to a nursing home or assisted-living facility after a surgical procedure by as much as 20-fold,[33]
- Increases the risk for falls and disability,
- Increases the risk ultimately for early death.[33]

TIPS TO REDUCE FRAILTY AND PROMOTE HEALTHY AGING

The severity of frailty can be reduced with appropriate interventions despite advanced age.[3] Some longitudinal population-based studies have shown that 8.3% to 17.9% of older adults actually improved their frailty levels, and some of them made frequent and dynamic transitions over time.[34–45] Herein are suggestions of some evidence-based interventions that can potentially mitigate the progression of frailty.

Exercise/Physical Activity

There is overwhelming evidence to support that physical activity/exercise consistently improves functional health, boosts energy balance, reduces the risk for frailty, and in fact, can potentially reverse the progression of frailty in older adults. In advanced age, physical activity is very effective at mitigating sarcopenia, restoring robustness, and preventing/delaying the development of disability and frailty.[46]

One of the largest and longest studies in this field is the "LIFE" (Lifestyle Interventions and Independence for Elders) study; a US-based multicenter randomized controlled trial in which 424 sedentary older adults at risk for disability were engaged in moderate-intensity physical activity or a successful aging intervention for an average of 1.2 years. The physical activity program consisted of a combination of walking at moderate intensity, resistance exercises, balance, stretching, and behavioral counseling. The successful aging educational program consisted of health education seminars and upper-extremity stretching exercises. Results from the LIFE study, over 1 year of follow-up, showed that the incidence of major mobility disability was significantly reduced with the physical activity program, a benefit that was fairly consistent across the board regardless of age, race, gender, and preexisting comorbidities.[47–49]

These results support the proposition that a physical exercise program, a combination of endurance and resistance exercises, is effective in preventing mobility disability and improving frailty in older adults.

The public health message from the Physical Activity Guidelines for Americans recommends that moderate physical activity should be performed for 30 minutes on most if not all days of the week (150–210 total minutes).[46]

Various forms of exercise are acceptable, including but not limited to, walking, resistance training, and aerobic exercise and can be modified into short intervals with multiple breaks to suit individual endurance capacity and comorbidities.

According to recent literature reviews, an optimal exercise intervention for frail older adults is performed at least 3 times a week with progressive moderate intensity for 30 to 45 minutes per session and for a duration of at least 5 months. The optimal type of exercise intervention is a multicomponent intervention, including aerobic exercise, strength training, balance, and flexibility.[50]

Physical exercise improves muscle sensitivity to protein or amino acid uptake, thus reducing the negative effect of anabolic resistance and sarcopenia while promoting buildup of muscle mass.

Exercise increases higher cerebral blood flow, which tends to promote overall cognitive performance. During exercise, "happy hormones," endorphins, are produced endogenously by the body to promote mood and mental health. Optimum mood and mental health help to increase individuals' motivation to stay compliant with interventions that reduce frailty and promote healthy aging.

The compelling evidence in favor of physical activity and exercise as an important core intervention to promote healthy aging has prompted the WHO to recommend engaging in regular physical activity throughout one's life.

Nutrition

There is strong evidence to show that the quality of the diet is inversely associated with the risk of becoming frail, which means that the better the quality of diet, the less the risk of becoming frail. A systematic review and metaanalysis published by Coelho-Junior and colleagues[51] suggest that a high consumption of dietary protein is inversely associated with frailty in older adults; a preestablished cutoff protein daily intake level of more than 1 g/kg of body weight was adopted by one of the studies.

The article by Lorenzo-López and colleagues[52] establishes the importance of consuming high dietary antioxidants, which are associated with a lower risk of developing frailty.

Altogether, both quantitative (energy intake) and qualitative (nutrient quality) factors of nutrition seem to play a key role in muscle building and risk reduction in developing sarcopenia and subsequent frailty in older adults.

Thus, high-calorie snacks and nutritional supplements are reasonable interventions in frail older adults who have lost weight and have poor nutrition, but more studies would be required before this can be made standard of care in prevention or reduction of frailty in nonmalnourished older adults.[53]

Optimum benefit of nutritional intervention in reducing frailty is best observed when combined with exercise.

Nutrition, Frailty, and Pressure Ulcers

It has been reported that frailty in the elderly combined with poor nutrition could put older adults at risk for compromised skin integrity and pressure sores.[54]

Because pressure ulcer is a geriatric syndrome that is now recognized as a disability by the Centers for Disease Control and Prevention, theoretically the coexistence of pressure ulcer and frailty combines to heighten the burden and risk for disability and potential early mortality.

Cognitive Stimulation

"Use it or lose it" is a popular slogan that is true with regards to frailty; it emphasizes the importance of keeping up with physical activities and cognitive stimulation to reduce frailty and promote wellness. If you do not use your muscles, they get weak; if you do not use your mind, it begins to fail.[55]

Keeping your mind active and your attitude optimistic potentially generates positive feelings, which translates into a lower risk for frailty in 1 study. "Staying socially connected with others and continuing to learn may also help." Durso[33] says. "Johns Hopkins research has found that these factors may explain why older volunteers who tutor in elementary schools sharpen their own thinking skills and improve their physical functioning too."

Sleep

We spend nearly one-third of our lives sleeping; thus, good quality sleep is an important aspect of wellness. Some emerging studies suggest that poor sleep is linked to inflammatory processes, which are associated with muscle loss and functional decline. Although the exact mechanism is unclear, several studies have shown a strong relationship between poor sleep and increased risk for frailty.

- In this prospective cohort study done by Ensrud and colleagues,[56] involving 2505 nonfrail men aged $\geq$67 years that were assessed subjectively (with questionnaires) and objectively with sleep parameters (from actigraphy and in-home overnight polysomnography), after an average of 3.4 years, it was concluded that among nonfrail older men, poor subjective sleep quality, greater nighttime wakefulness, and greater nocturnal hypoxemia were independently associated with a higher odds of frailty or death at follow-up, whereas excessive daytime sleepiness, greater nighttime wakefulness, severe sleep apnea, and greater nocturnal hypoxemia were independently associated with an increased risk of mortality.
- In an observational study involving 2889 women with a mean age of 83.5 years, who participated in the 2002 to 2004 examination of the Study of Osteoporotic Fractures, the subjects wore actigraphs, which measured sleep variables like total sleep time, hours awake after sleep onset during the night, and daytime napping behavior. Neuromuscular performance measurements included gait speed, chair stands, and grip strength. Functional limitations were assessed as self-reported difficulty with one or more of 6 instrumental activities of daily living (IADL). After fully adjusted, this study showed that objectively measured poorer sleep was associated with worse physical function.[57]
- In another prospective cohort study involving 817 women with a mean age of 82.4 at baseline who wore wrist actigraphy to objectively measure sleep parameters, functional status indices like IADL, grip strength, and gait speed were measured at baseline and after 5 years, Findings indicate that shorter "sleep duration," greater "wake after sleep onset," and lower "sleep efficiency" are risk factors for functional/physical decline in older women.[58]
- The Osteoporotic Fractures in Men Research Group study involving 2862 community-dwelling men demonstrated that greater sleep fragmentation and hypoxia are associated with poorer physical function in older men.[59]

Therefore, there is compelling evidence to suggest that poor sleep impacts negatively on key components of frailty. Future research is needed to identify the underlying mechanisms for the association between poor sleep and functional decline.

Social Interaction

There is growing evidence to support the benefits of social relationships and interactions on general health/wellness. It is true that recent findings from population studies have demonstrated the protective role of social relations on various health outcomes, including dementia, depression, recovery from acute illness, survival, morbidity, and well-being.[60]

"Social relations" is generally defined as the individuals whom one has an interpersonal relationship with. Important components of social relations include *number* of social relations, the *frequency* of seeing other people, the *diversity* of social relations, and *the reciprocity* of social relations.[60]

Social interaction can be achieved not only by face-to- face encounters but also by voice telephone calls, face-time telephone calls, skyping, and other technologically enabled mediums of communication.

A longitudinal cohort study done by Buchman and colleagues[61] involving 906 persons with a mean follow-up of 4.9 years showed that less frequent participation in social activities is associated with more rapid rate of motor function decline in old age.

In a study done by Avlund and colleagues, using data on 651 nondisabled 75-year-old persons who later had a 5-year follow-up, results showed that, in men, no weekly telephone contact was related to functional decline and mortality. Among women, less than weekly telephone contact, no membership in a retirement club, and not sewing for others were significantly related to functional decline and mortality.

The results stress the importance of social relations in the prevention of functional decline in older adults.[60]

Management of Polypharmacy

There is emerging evidence to support that a reduction of polypharmacy could be an important intervention to prevent and manage frailty.

Gutiérrez-Valencia and colleagues[62] conducted the first known systematic review analyzing the available evidence on the relationship between frailty and polypharmacy in older adults.

A total of 25 publications were included, and the analyses demonstrated a significant association between an increased number of medications and frailty. Although the actual causal relationship is unclear and appears to be bidirectional, the analysis of published data suggests that polypharmacy could be a major contributor to the development of frailty and should be addressed when present in frail or prefrail older adults.[62]

The US Preventive Service Task Force recommendations for management of frailty includes a comprehensive care plan that should address polypharmacy, the management of sarcopenia, the treatable causes of weight loss, and the causes of exhaustion (depression, anemia, hypotension, hypothyroidism, and B12 deficiency) (strong recommendation). All persons with frailty should receive social support as needed to address unmet needs and encourage adherence to a comprehensive care plan (strong recommendation). First-line therapy for the management of frailty should include a multicomponent physical activity program with a resistance-based training component (strong recommendation). Protein/caloric supplementation is recommended when weight loss or undernutrition is present (conditional recommendation). No recommendation was given for systematic additional therapies, such as cognitive therapy, problem-solving therapy, vitamin D supplementation, and hormone-based treatment. Pharmacologic treatment was not a recommended therapy for the treatment of frailty.[14]

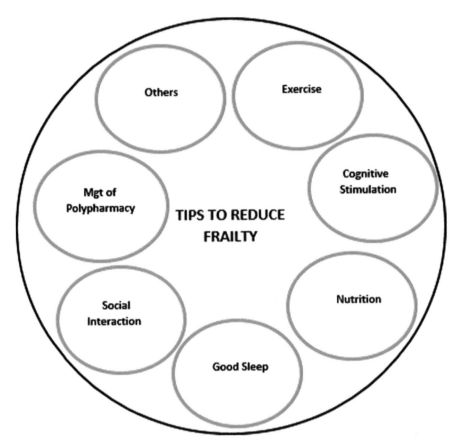

Fig. 7. Multicomponent frailty intervention model.

Other potentially beneficial interventions include (but are not limited to) management of mood disorder, stress management to promote healthy aging (this will be discussed in a separate article), optimizing management of chronic diseases, and smoking cessation. All of these strategies are generally acceptable to promote wellness, but evidence in favor of these interventions with specific regards to frailty is still fairly limited at this time.

SUMMARY

Frailty is an important concept in geriatric medicine and is increasingly considered "the hallmark" geriatric syndrome. It is regarded as a precursor to many other geriatric syndromes, including (but not limited to) falls, osteoporosis, fractures, failure to thrive, incontinence, and even delirium.[3]

An older adult may be considered frail if 3 or more of these following criteria apply:

1. "Shrinking": unintentional loss of 10 or more pounds in the past year.
2. Feeling weak: trouble standing without assistance or have reduced grip strength.
3. Feeling exhausted: it takes a big effort to do most things or one cannot get going 3 or more days most weeks.

4. Low activity level: this includes difficulty with household chores, hobbies, or exercise.
5. Slow walking: if it takes more than 6 or 7 seconds to walk 15 feet.[33]

Because frailty is a multisystemic syndrome, it will likely require a multidomain approach to effectively treat/manage frailty. This approach may include (but is not limited to) exercise, optimum nutrition, cognitive stimulation activities, sleep, social interaction, management of and polypharmacy, among others. Multicomponent interventions, as shown in **Fig. 7**, are considered more effective than monocomponent interventions in combating frailty to promote healthy aging.

Clearly, there is robust evidence to suggest that a multidomain intervention that combines physical therapy, cognitive stimulation, nutritional intervention, sleep, and social interaction improves frailty and functional status; more studies will be needed to include other wellness interventions like stress and mood management, such as yoga/mindfulness, geriatric assessment, management of chronic illness, and perhaps specific pharmacologic strategies.

It is expected that more evidence-based studies in these areas will potentially provide a premise to develop a solid broad-spectrum multicomponent care model that would serve as standard of care geared toward reducing frailty to promote healthy aging.

DISCLOSURE

The authors have nothing to disclose.

REFERENCES

1. Kojima G, Liljas AEM, Iliffe S. Frailty syndrome: implications and challenges for health care policy. Risk Manag Healthc Policy 2019;12:23–30.
2. Ediev DM. Life Expectancy in Developed Countries is Higher Than Conventionally Estimated. Implications from Improved Measurement of Human Longevity. Population Ageing 2011;4:5. https://doi.org/10.1007/s12062-011-9040-x.
3. Walston JD. Frailty. Available at: https://www.uptodate.com/contents/frailty. Accessed September 7, 2019.
4. Fried LP, Tangen CM, Walston J, et al. Frailty in older adults: evidence for phenotype. J Gerontol A Biol Sci Med Sci 2001;56:M146.
5. Rothenberg KA, Stern JR, George EL, et al. Association of frailty and postoperative complications with unplanned readmissions after elective outpatient surgery. JAMA Netw Open 2019;2(5):e194330.
6. Elizabeth W. Markson. Functional, social, and psychological disability as causes of loss of weight and independence in older community-living people. Clin Geriatr Med 1997;13:639–52.
7. Xue QL. The frailty syndrome: definition and natural history. Clin Geriatr Med 2011;27(1):1–15.
8. Collard RM, Boter H, Schoevers RA, et al. Prevalence of frailty in community-dwelling older persons: a systematic review. J Am Geriatr Soc 2012;60(8):1487–92.
9. Handforth C, Clegg A, Young C, et al. The prevalence and outcomes of frailty in older cancer patients: a systematic review. Ann Oncol 2015;26(6):1091–101.
10. Kojima G. Prevalence of frailty in end-stage renal disease: a systematic review and meta-analysis. Int Urol Nephrol 2017;49(11):1989–97.

11. Denfeld QE, Winters-Stone K, Mudd JO, et al. The prevalence of frailty in heart failure: a systematic review and meta-analysis. Int J Cardiol 2017;236:283–9.
12. Kojima G, Liljas A, Iliffe S, et al. Prevalence of frailty in mild to moderate Alzheimer's disease: a systematic review and meta-analysis. Curr Alzheimer Res 2017;14(12):1256–63.
13. Kojima G. Prevalence of frailty in nursing homes: a systematic review and meta-analysis. J Am Med Dir Assoc 2015;16(11):940–5.
14. Dent E, Morley JE, Cruz-Jentoft AJ, et al. Physical frailty: ICFSR international clinical practice guidelines for identification and management. J Nutr Health Aging 2019;23(9):771–87.
15. Cappola AR, Xue QL, Ferrucci L, et al. Insulin-like growth factor I and interleukin-6 contribute synergistically to disability and mortality in older women. J Clin Endocrinol Metab 2003;88:2019.
16. Schmidt M, Naumann H, Weidler C, et al. Inflammation and sex hormone metabolism. Ann N Y Acad Sci 2006;1069:236.
17. Varadhan R, Walston J, Cappola AR, et al. Higher levels and blunted diurnal variation of cortisol in frail older women. J Gerontol A Biol Sci Med Sci 2008;63:190.
18. Ershler WB. Biological interactions of aging and anemia: a focus on cytokines. J Am Geriatr Soc 2003;51:S18.
19. Leng S, Chaves P, Koenig K, et al. Serum interleukin-6 and hemoglobin as physiological correlates in the geriatric syndrome of frailty: a pilot study. J Am Geriatr Soc 2002;50:1268.
20. Puts MT, Visser M, Twisk JW, et al. Endocrine and inflammatory markers as predictors of frailty. Clin Endocrinol (Oxf) 2005;63:403.
21. Kaditz E, Johansen K, Cuenoud H, et al. University of Massachusetts medical school homeostenosis. The portal for online geriatric learning. vol. 22. 2019. Available at: Portal of Geriatrics Online Education -see link https://www.pogoe.org/image/9504.
22. Woods NF, LaCroix AZ, Gray SL, et al. Frailty: emergence and consequences in women aged 65 and older in the Women's Health Initiative Observational Study. J Am Geriatr Soc 2005;53:1321.
23. Cawthon PM, Marshall LM, Michael Y, et al. Frailty in older men: prevalence, progression, and relationship with mortality. J Am Geriatr Soc 2007;55:1216.
24. Bandeen-Roche K, Seplaki CL, Huang J, et al. Frailty in older adults: a nationally representative profile in the United States. J Gerontol A Biol Sci Med Sci 2015;70:1427.
25. Lakey SL, LaCroix AZ, Gray SL, et al. Antidepressant use, depressive symptoms, and incident frailty in women aged 65 and older from the Women's Health Initiative Observational Study. J Am Geriatr Soc 2012;60:854.
26. Evenhuis HM, Hermans H, Hilgenkamp TI, et al. Frailty and disability in older adults with intellectual disabilities: results from the Healthy Ageing and Intellectual Disability Study. J Am Geriatr Soc 2012;60:934.
27. Lee L, Heckman G, Molnar FJ. Frailty: identifying elderly patients at high risk of poor outcomes. Can Fam Physician 2015;61(3):227–31.
28. Rockwood K, Mitnitski A. Frailty in relation to the accumulation of deficits. J Gerontol A Biol Sci Med Sci 2007;62:722.
29. Ensrud KE, Ewing SK, Taylor BC, et al. Comparison of 2 frailty indexes for prediction of falls, disability, fractures, and death in older women. Arch Intern Med 2008;168:382.
30. Fritz S, Lusardi M. White paper: "walking speed: the sixth vital sign". J Geriatr Phys Ther 2009;32(2):46–9.

31. Abellan van Kan G, Rolland Y, Andrieu S, et al. Gait speed at usual pace as a predictor of adverse outcomes in community-dwelling older people an international academy on nutrition and aging (IANA) task force. J Nutr Health Aging 2009 Dec;13(10):881–9.

32. Liu M, DuMontier C, Murillo A. Gait speed, grip strength and clinical outcomes in older patients with hematologic malignancies. Blood 2019;134(4):374–82.

33. Durso S. Available at: https://www.hopkinsmedicine.org/health/wellness-and-prevention/stay-strong-four-ways-to-beat-the-frailty-risk. Accessed October 5, 2019.

34. Ma L, Tang Z, Zhang L, et al. Prevalence of frailty and associated factors in the community-dwelling population of China. J Am Geriatr Soc 2018;66(3):559–64.

35. Kehler DS, Ferguson T, Stammers AN, et al. Prevalence of frailty in Canadians 18–79 years old in the Canadian Health Measures Survey. BMC Geriatr 2017;17(1):28.

36. Payne CF, Wade A, Kabudula CW, et al. Prevalence and correlates of frailty in an older rural African population: findings from the HAALSI cohort study. BMC Geriatr 2017;17(1):293.

37. Lewis EG, Coles S, Howorth K, et al. The prevalence and characteristics of frailty by frailty phenotype in rural Tanzania. BMC Geriatr 2018;18(1):283.

38. Kojima G, Taniguchi Y, Iliffe S, et al. Transitions between frailty states among community-dwelling older people: a systematic review and meta-analysis. Ageing Res Rev 2019;50:81–8.

39. Espinoza SE, Jung I, Hazuda H. Frailty transitions in the San Antonio longitudinal study of aging. J Am Geriatr Soc 2012;60(4):652–60.

40. Lanziotti Azevedo da Silva S, Campos Cavalcanti Maciel Á, de Sousa Máximo Pereira L, et al. Transition patterns of frailty syndrome in community-dwelling elderly individuals: a longitudinal study. J Frailty Aging 2015;4(2):50–5.

41. Lee JS, Auyeung TW, Leung J, et al. Transitions in frailty states among community-living older adults and their associated factors. J Am Med Dir Assoc 2014;15(4):281–6.

42. Liu ZY, Wei YZ, Wei LQ, et al. Frailty transitions and types of death in Chinese older adults: a population-based cohort study. Clin Interv Aging 2018;13:947–56.

43. Pollack LR, Litwack-Harrison S, Cawthon PM, et al. Patterns and predictors of frailty transitions in older men: the Osteoporotic Fractures in Men Study. J Am Geriatr Soc 2017;65(11):2473–9.

44. Trevisan C, Veronese N, Maggi S, et al. Factors influencing transitions between frailty states in elderly adults: the Progetto Veneto Anziani Longitudinal Study. J Am Geriatr Soc 2017;65(1):179–84.

45. Gill TM, Gahbauer EA, Allore HG, et al. Transitions between frailty states among community-living older persons. Arch Intern Med 2006;166(4):418–23.

46. Marzetti E, Calvani R, Tosato M, et al. Physical activity and exercise as countermeasures to physical frailty and sarcopenia. Aging Clin Exp Res 2017;29:35. Available at: http://health.gov/paguidelines/pdf/paguide.pdf.

47. Pahor M, Guralnik JM, Ambrosius WT, et al. Effect of structured physical activity on prevention of major mobility disability in older adults: the LIFE study randomized clinical trial. JAMA 2014;311:2387–96.

48. Pahor M, Blair SN, Espeland M, et al. Effects of a physical activity intervention on measures of physical performance: results of the Lifestyle Interventions and Independence for Elders Pilot (LIFE-P) study. J Gerontol A Biol Sci Med Sci 2006;61:1157–65.

49. Guralnik JM, Simonsick EM, Ferrucci L, et al. A short physical performance battery assessing lower extremity function: association with self-reported disability and prediction of mortality and nursing home admission. J Gerontol 1994;49: M85–94.

50. Dedeyne L, Deschodt M, Verschueren S, et al. Effects of multi-domain interventions in (pre)frail elderly on frailty, functional, and cognitive status: a systematic review. Dove Press 2017;12:873–96.

51. Coelho-Junior HJ, Rodrigues B, Uchida M, et al. Low protein intake is associated with frailty in older adults: a systematic review and meta-analysis of observational studies. MDPI Nutrients 2018;10(9):1334.

52. Lorenzo-López L, Maseda A, de Labra C, et al. Nutritional determinants of frailty in older adults: a systematic review pubmed.gov. BMC Geriatr 2017;17(1):108.

53. Wallace JI, Schwartz RS. Involuntary weight loss in elderly outpatients: recognition, etiologies, and treatment. Clin Geriatr Med 1997;13(4):717–35.

54. Hwa Hsu CC, et al. Poster session. Presented at: AANP 2015. June 10-14; New Orleans. Available at: https://www.clinicaladvisor.com/home/meeting-coverage/aanp-2015-annual-meeting/factors-leading-to-frailty-in-elderly-and-its-complications-identified/. Accessed November 2, 2019.

55. Morley John E, Sandford AM. Editorial: screening for sarcopenia. J Nutr Health Aging 2019;23(9):768–70.

56. Ensrud KE, Blackwell TL, Ancoli-Israel S, et al. Sleep disturbances and risk of frailty and mortality in older men. Sleep Med 2012;13(10):1217–25.

57. Goldman SE, Stone KL, Ancoli-Israel S, et al. Poor sleep is associated with poorer physical performance and greater functional limitations in older women. Sleep 2007;30(10):1317–24.

58. Spira AP, Covinsky K, Rebok GW, et al. Poor sleep quality and functional decline in older women. J Am Geriatr Soc 2012;60(6):1092–8.

59. Dam TT, Ewing S, Ancoli-Israel S, et al. Osteoporotic Fractures in Men Research Group. Association between sleep and physical function in older men: the osteoporotic fractures in men sleep study. J Am Geriatr Soc 2008;56(9):1665–73.

60. Avlund K, Lund R, Holstein BE, et al. The impact of structural and functional characteristics of social relations as determinants of functional decline. J Gerontol B Psychol Sci Soc Sci 2004;59(1):S44–51. https://doi.org/10.1093/geronb/59.1. S44. Available at:.

61. Buchman AS, Boyle PA, Wilson RS, et al. Association between late-life social activity and motor decline in older adults. Arch Intern Med 2009;169(12):1139–46.

62. Gutiérrez-Valencia M, Izquierdo M, Cesari M, et al. The relationship between frailty and polypharmacy in older people: a systematic reviewBr. J Clin Pharmacol 2018;84(7):1432–44.

Addressing Obesity to Promote Healthy Aging

Meredith N. Roderka, BS[a], Sadhana Puri, BS[b], John A. Batsis, MD, FTOS[a,b,c,d,e,*]

KEYWORDS

- Obesity • Older adults • Healthy aging

KEY POINTS

- This article reviews epidemiology of obesity including increase in prevalence, race/ethnicity, and socioeconomic disparities.
- Consequences of obesity in older adults include falls, cognitive decline, fractures, quality of life, disability, and nursing home admissions.
- There are specific benefits to intentional weight loss on physical function and comorbidity but also key risks to muscle and bone loss that need to be understood.
- Health care professionals should encourage older adults with obesity to try to implement healthy lifestyle behaviors that include exercise and diet routine.

INTRODUCTION

The population worldwide is aging and is not immune to the changing prevalence of obesity (**Fig. 1**). Older adults with obesity are at risk for adverse events, including functional decline, institutionalization, and mortality. Other consequences of obesity and changes in body composition with aging are an increased risk of falls, fractures, reduced quality of life (QoL), and cognitive decline. This article describes the epidemiology of obesity, its geriatric-specific consequences, and the benefits and risks of intentional weight loss (**Fig. 2**).

Dr. Batsis receives funding from the National Institute on Aging of the National Institutes of Health under Award Number K23AG051681. The content is solely the responsibility of the authors and does not necessarily represent the official views of the National Institutes of Health.
[a] Section of Weight & Wellness, Department of Medicine, Dartmouth-Hitchcock Medical Center, 1 Medical Center Drive, Lebanon, NH 03756, USA; [b] Geisel School of Medicine, 1 Rope Ferry Road, Hanover, NH 03755, USA; [c] The Dartmouth Institute for Health & Clinical Practice, 1 Medical Center Drive, Lebanon, NH 03756, USA; [d] Dartmouth Centers for Health and Aging Hitchcock Loop Road, Lebanon, NH 03766, USA; [e] Section of General Internal Medicine, Dartmouth-Hitchcock Medical Center, 1 Medical Center Drive, Lebanon, NH 03756, USA
* Corresponding author. Section of General Internal Medicine, Dartmouth-Hitchcock Medical Center, 1 Medical Center Drive, Lebanon, NH 03756.
E-mail address: john.batsis@gmail.com

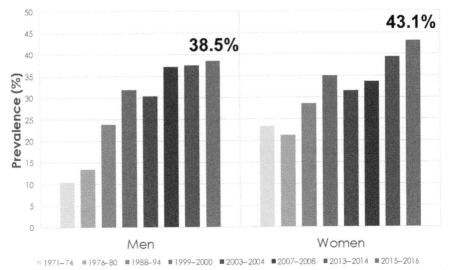

Fig. 1. Population with obesity in the United States. (*Data from* the National Health and Nutrition Examination Survey demonstrating the changing demographics of older adults.)

EPIDEMIOLOGY OF OBESITY IN OLDER ADULTS

It is projected that more than 83.7 million people in the United States will be older than 65 years in the year 2050.[1] This demographic shift is largely caused by an increase in baby boomers and improved medical care, all which have led to an increase in life expectancy.[1] The most recent National Health and Nutrition Examination Survey data highlight an obesity prevalence of approximately 41% in adults aged 60 and older,[2] which leads to consequences resulting in impaired physical function,[3] decreased QoL, institutionalization,[4] and death.[5]

Rates of obesity in older adults have also increased worldwide,[6] with rates tripling over the past 40 years.[7] Drivers of this epidemic include changes in the global food system, an increased intake of energy-dense foods and sedentary work, expanding urbanization, changes in transportation modalities, and the interactions of biologic and environmental factors. There are important disparities observed in obesity rates in older adults including race/ethnicity,[8] rural/urban,[2] and socioeconomic status (SES).[9] In 2007 to 2010, Hispanic men aged 75 and older had a higher prevalence of obesity (27.9%) when compared with non-Hispanic White men (26.4%),[10] with different rates observed in women (49.4% in non-Hispanic Black, 30.2% in Hispanic, and 27.5% in non-Hispanic White).[10] In the United States, obesity prevalence was higher in rural than in urban residents.[9] SES influences the development of obesity in developed and low-income countries.[11] Few studies demonstrate associations between SES and obesity in older adults. Individuals aged greater than or equal to 50 years with financial hardship in the EPIC-Norfolk study were at higher risk for obesity irrespective of education, social class, or home ownership.[12]

CHANGES IN BODY COMPOSITION

Aging is associated with body composition changes, including loss of skeletal muscle mass and redistribution of fat to the abdominal area and visceral organs. With age, there is a gradual increase in body fat, specifically visceral adipose tissue,[13] a trend continuing until extreme old age when fat mass may decrease.[14] Abdominal fat

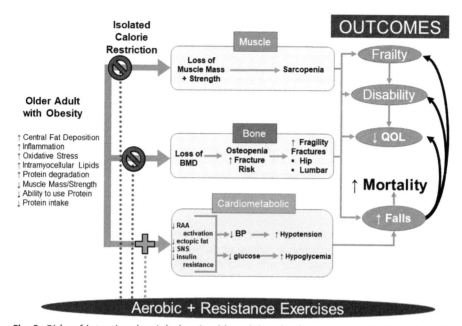

Fig. 2. Risks of intentional weight loss in older adults. This figure represents the major risks associated with isolated calorie-restricted, diet-induced weight loss on muscle, bone, and the cardiometabolic system and their impact on key outcomes of frailty, disability, quality of life, falls, and mortality. The interrelationships between these elements are presented through the *arrows*. Elements of the underlying pathophysiologic processes in aging in the older adult with obesity are presented. Aerobic and resistance exercises coupled with diet-induced weight loss mitigate the loss of muscle mass and strength, and bone mineral density (indicated by *red dotted line* and *prohibition symbol*). This combination also stimulates enhancement of elements of the cardiometabolic system leading to improvements in glucose homeostasis and blood pressure, requiring providers to be cognizant of relative hypotension and hypoglycemia (indicated by *green dotted line* and *plus symbol*). BMD, bone mineral density; BP, blood pressure; QOL, quality of life; RAA, renin, angiotensin, aldosterone; SNS, sympathetic nervous system. (*From* DiMilia PR, Mittman AC, Batsis JA. Benefit-to-risk balance of weight loss interventions in older adults with obesity. Curr Diab Rep. 2019;19(11):114; with permission.)

redistribution significantly contributes to insulin sensitivity and metabolic syndrome[15] and is a correlate of cardiometabolic disease.[16] Visceral fat promotes intramuscular fat infiltration, which leads to proinflammatory cytokine production, ultimately contributing to reduced muscle and physical function.[17]

As muscle mass declines with age,[18] the amount of available insulin-responsive tissue drops, which may also lead to insulin resistance. Starting at age 30, there is approximately a 20% to 40% decrease in muscle mass by age 70, which may lead to sarcopenia,[19] the age-related loss of muscle mass and strength.[20] The Health, Aging and Body Composition Study noted a loss of muscle mass was associated with a decline in strength in older adults,[21] but the decline in strength was more rapid than the loss of mass, suggesting a decline in muscle quality.[22] Changes in skeletal muscle mass and function is critically important because it affects older adults' mobility and function.

Although body mass index (BMI) is a simple and inexpensive method for assessing obesity, it lacks sensitivity and may underestimate adiposity in older adults.[18] This is, in part, caused by its inability to discriminate between subcutaneous and visceral fat, and failing to account for muscle and bone mass. In contrast, waist circumference easily approximates increased intra-abdominal fat[23] with its sensitivity exceeding that of BMI, and is strongly associated with an increased morbidity risk.[24] Despite such limitations, BMI is valuable at the population level by allowing health professionals to make comparisons across time, regions, and subgroups.

CONSEQUENCES OF OBESITY

Consequences of obesity include cardiometabolic dysfunction, arthritis, pulmonary, urinary incontinence, cataracts, and cancer.[25] Specific to older adults include an increased risk of falls, cognitive decline, QoL, and disability, which are reviewed next.[18]

Falls

Obesity negatively impacts balance and increases postural sway,[26] predisposing to falling and negatively impacting activities of daily living.[27] Among middle-aged and older adults, obesity is associated with a higher prevalence of falls and stumbling during ambulation.[28] The prevalence of falls differs in men and women, with middle-aged women at a particularly higher risk,[29] which may be caused by an increased rate of trip-related falls.[30] This has implications in sarcopenic obesity; in older men with obesity, for instance, the loss of muscle mass is associated with an increased risk of falls,[31] with rates higher in this population.[32] Participants with obesity that fall have a higher prevalence of pain and inactivity than fallers of a healthy weight.[28]

Fractures

The association between hip fractures and obesity is less understood with conflicting associations.[33] A prospective population-based study of sarcopenic obese men found a high risk of fracture.[31] Weight loss leads to loss of bone density. Intentional weight loss was strongly associated with an increased risk of hip fracture. The pathophysiology associated with such fractures and whether obesity impacts bone quality is unclear and requires further investigation.[33]

Quality of Life

The presence of obesity in older adults negatively impacts QoL, in part caused by the loss of physical function that accompanies obesity.[34] Older obese adults were found to have a lower health-related QoL in the Medical Expenditure Panel Survey.[18] A study examining the relationship between BMI and QoL among adults aged greater than or equal to 60 years old[35] found that overweight older women were more likely to have lower scores and overweight older men were less likely to have low visual analog scale compared with normal BMI. Gaining an understanding of the differences in QoL in older obese adults could be helpful in tailoring specific interventions.

Cognitive Impairment

Several studies have explored the relationship between obesity and cognitive impairment.[36–38] Overweight and obesity demonstrated lower neuropsychological test scores than individuals with a normal BMI. Bischof and Park[39] explored whether obesity in midlife or later life placed older adults at greater risk for cognitive decline and found that midlife obesity increased the risk for cognitive decline in late-life. Others demonstrated that conventional care plus nutritional counseling (vs conventional care) in obese patients greater than 60 years led to significant weight loss and improved global cognition, memory, semantic fluency, and Wisconsin categories.[37] Even a diet, exercise, and diet-exercise intervention in frail older obese adults age greater than or equal to 65 led to improved modified mini-mental status scores, trail making, and word fluency tests compared with control subjects at 1 year.[38] In contrast, the intensive lifestyle arm in Look-AHEAD[40] found no significant difference in the prevalence of cognitive impairment compared with control subjects.[36] There is promise that improved diet-exercise may positively impact cognition; further efficacy studies are needed.

Disability

Disability is one of the most devastating consequences in older obese adults that leads to higher utilization,[41] institutionalization,[42] and death.[43] Several factors promote the development of disablement process, from a mechanical and inflammatory standpoint. Body fat redistribution promotes intramuscular fat infiltration leading to a vicious cycle of proinflammatory cytokine production and contributing to reduced muscle function (**Fig. 3**).[17] Inflammatory-based lipotoxicity reduces the potential of muscular regeneration leading to muscle fibrosis,[44] promotes insulin resistance, and negatively impacts muscle strength.[17] Such tissue damage inhibits the regeneration of muscle mass in those with sarcopenic obesity that negatively impacts physical function. For example, greater muscle fat infiltration was associated with an increased risk of mobility limitation.[45] A meta-analysis found that a BMI greater than or equal to 30 kg/m² with low muscle strength in older adults, and not low muscle mass, was associated with functional decline.[45] Persons with sarcopenic obesity have difficulty ascending and descending the stairs.[46] Applying newer sarcopenia definitions, the presence of sarcopenic obesity resulted in an increased risk of frailty, activity of daily living disability, and instrumental activity of daily living disability.[47] Data from the

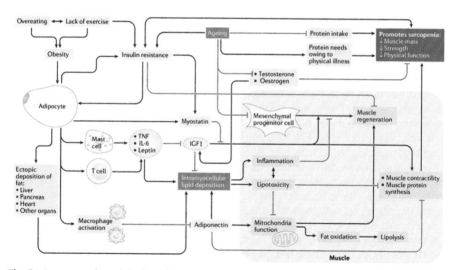

Fig. 3. A proposed model of mechanisms leading to sarcopenic obesity. The proposed interplay between adipose and muscle tissue, which is believed to contribute to the development of sarcopenic obesity, is shown. The *black lines* are stimulatory, and *red lines with flat ends* indicate inhibition. IGF1, insulin-like growth factor 1; IL, interleukin; TNF, tumor necrosis factor. (*From* Batsis JA, Villareal DT. Sarcopenic obesity in older adults: aetiology, epidemiology and treatment strategies. Nat Rev Endocrinol. 2018;14(9):513–37; with permission.)

Osteoarthritis Initiative also showed that a combination of low knee extensor strength and high BMI was associated with reduced gait speed, a lower degree of physical function, and decreased self-reported health status.[48] Considerable evidence exists to suggest that sarcopenia and obesity is strongly associated with reduced physical function in older adults.

Nursing Home Admission

Older obese adults are at a higher risk for nursing home admission. A review suggested that obesity early in life is a risk factor for future admission,[42] even for middle-aged persons.[49] Separately, there was a greater rate of nursing home admission in Whites with obesity compared with a normal BMI but no relationship in Blacks.[50] Between 1992 and 2002, the proportion of newly admitted residents with obesity to nursing homes rose from 15% to 25%.[51] The distribution of residents with obesity was also unequal across different facilities, ranging from 0% to 40%, highlighting the inability of nursing homes to accommodate such residents.[51] The increased number of obese patients admitted to nursing homes can also impact the institution's ability to accommodate such patients. Patient size was a barrier to admission,[52] but also led to increased time to accomplish care needs.[53] Nursing home administrators reported inadequate staffing for the care of morbidly obese residents in 31% of nursing homes and also reported concerns about having the proper equipment for individuals with obesity in 68% of nursing homes.[52]

OBESITY PARADOX

A major challenge for clinical providers has been whether to recommend weight loss interventions in older adults. This controversy, coined "the obesity paradox," stems, in part, from the inverse correlation between higher adiposity and mortality observed from several epidemiologic studies; data have been strongest among older adults.

Previous studies demonstrated that obesity is associated with increased survival in those with established cardiovascular disease (CVD).[54] There has also been support for the paradox in the context of type 2 diabetes, suggesting lower mortality in patients with type 2 diabetes and obesity than in normal or lower weight patients.[55] The paradox has been described in chronic obstructive pulmonary disease and in nursing home residents.[56] There are strong critics who believe the term "paradox" is misleading because it was derived from biased observational studies.[57] Several arguments dispel this paradox. Previous studies do not differentiate between unintentional weight loss associated with chronic illness and intentional weight loss.[57,58] The potential for bias increases with older age as the presence of chronic diseases accumulate, possibly explaining why this paradox is so prominent in older individuals.[58] Possible confounders are not accounted for (smoking, cardiorespiratory fitness, or socioeconomic variables).[57] Last, mortality studies have stratified by smoking status, which is associated with a lower BMI.[58]

A key study refuting the obesity paradox analyzed the association between BMI and lifetime risk of CVD. The study design accounted for measurement, selection, and survival bias and variable follow-up times by stratifying the risk for non-CVD death by age, sex, and BMI strata to observe the relationship between BMI and risk of mortality from CVD in an isolated fashion. Overweight and obesity were associated with a significantly increased risk for CVD, and obesity was associated with a shorter lifespan and a greater proportion of life lived with CVD. Incident CVD among middle-aged men and women with morbid obesity was accelerated by 7.5 and 7.1 years compared with middle-aged men and women with normal BMI. Men and women with normal BMI lived an average of 5.6 and 2.0 years, respectively, longer than those with morbid obesity. Future studies can learn from and build on the methods of this study.

BENEFITS OF WEIGHT LOSS IN OLDER ADULTS

Guidelines support the role of intentional weight loss in older adults in improving physical function.[3] Clinicians need to individualize health promotion efforts and be aware of specific adverse events in this at-risk population. We briefly describe the risks/benefits of diet/exercise-induced weight loss in older adults because there is a limited evidence base for pharmacotherapy and bariatric surgery. Other benefits are outlined in a recent review.[59]

A review of weight loss interventions in older adults[60] found a greater degree of weight loss in groups with a dietary component than in those with exercise alone. Exercise alone led to improved physical function and increased fat-free mass without significant weight loss. A combined diet/exercise approach led to the greatest improvement in physical performance and QoL, mitigating the reduction in muscle and bone mass observed in diet-only arms. More recently, a review assessed the impact of treating obesity in older persons[61] and found that lifestyle interventions resulted in similar weight loss efficacy in older and younger people. Positive effects were observed on such outcomes as physical function and cardiovascular health. Weight loss led to improved QoL of older adults in a 6-month study.[62] Weight loss plus the addition of any form of exercise (aerobic or resistance) has produced an improvement in QoL scores beyond those observed in the weight loss–only conditions.[63] These findings suggest the importance in counseling patients in achieving their weight loss goals to help them improve their overall QoL.

Recent trials demonstrate the synergy of diet and exercise on improving physical function in older obese adults more than either separately.[64] Peak oxygen consumption increased more in the calorie restriction with aerobic/resistance training and diet-aerobic groups than in the diet-resistance group alone. Strength was higher in the diet-aerobic/resistance and resistance groups alone than in the aerobic group. Lean mass and hip bone mineral density decreased less in the diet-aerobic/resistance and resistance groups than in the aerobic group. Participants in LOOK-Ahead had improved gait speed greater than 4-m- and 400-m-walk tests and higher short performance physical battery scores over control subjects.[65]

A meta-analysis showed that caloric restriction plus aerobic and resistance exercise helped preserve fat-free mass in older adults, supporting the role of these strategies in the treatment of sarcopenic obesity.[66] A randomized trial of a dietary intervention in older obese adults and hypertension resulted in a mean 3.5-kg reduction in weight and a decreased need for antihypertensive medications by 30%.[67] Another study found that weight loss via diet and exercise effectively reduced pain and improved function and QoL in older adults with knee osteoarthritis in comparison with diet or exercise alone.[68] Hence, the optimal approach to improve physical function in older adults with obesity is a multicomponent, caloric restriction combined with aerobic and resistance program.

Protein supplementation has been proposed to reduce the potential weight loss–induced muscle loss. Consumption throughout the day can reduce the likelihood of weight loss–induced sarcopenia by stimulating muscle protein synthesis. The PROT-Age group recommends 1.0 to 1.1 g/kg protein per day in divided doses, acknowledging that a "one size fits all protein recommendation" fails to account for the complex physiologic changes of aging.[69] Of three studies evaluating the effects of high- versus low-protein diets in older adults with obesity,[70] only one study[70] demonstrated a significant benefit of a high-protein diet versus normal-protein diet on the short performance physical battery. Although weight loss was achieved at a comparable level in both groups, there were discrepancies in the age and sex of participants.[70] Future studies are critically needed.

RISKS OF WEIGHT LOSS

There are inherent risks that health care providers should be mindful of when counseling patients. Recognizing sarcopenia in the context of obesity is important[71] because reduction in caloric intake may lead to reduced adipose tissue, but also loss of muscle mass. Caloric restriction alone as a means of weight loss can increase the risk of sarcopenia, bone loss, and musculoskeletal injury in older adults.[48,59]

We advise caloric restriction should be coupled with resistance-based exercises. In one systematic review, unopposed calorie restriction without resistance training led to the loss of muscle mass and handgrip strength of up to 4.6% and 1.7 kg, respectively.[72] Diet-only interventions without exercise in older frail adults led to a marked loss of lean mass compared with diet-exercise, where the loss of lean mass was partially mitigated.[64] A review evaluating the effects of energy restriction on adults with a BMI greater than or equal to 25 kg/m^2 showed that 81% of caloric restriction groups and 39% of caloric restriction with exercise led to greater than or equal to 15% loss in fat-free mass, whereas exercise alone only led to modest loss in fat-free mass. Look-AHEAD participants showed significant reductions in total skeletal muscle mass in the intensive lifestyle group compared with control subjects.[73] In a 4-month trial, overweight and older adults in the caloric restriction group experienced a significant decrease in fat-free mass in contrast to the caloric restriction and exercise group. Recommendations for weight loss in older obese adults that allow for fat-free mass preservation include 150 minutes of aerobic exercise/week, 2 to 3 days of weight-bearing exercises/wk, protein supplementation 1.0 to 1.2 g/kg/d, and 1000 IU vitamin D or high-dose supplementation (if necessary).[59]

Calorie restriction alone has also demonstrated reduced bone-mineral density. Soltani and coworkers[74] reviewed 32 randomized trials in adults greater than or equal to 18 years and found that weight loss significantly led to reductions in hip and lumbar spine bone density. Hip bone density decline with weight loss was more pronounced in participants with obesity.[74] A 1-year study of older adults with obesity were randomized to caloric restriction, exercise, calorie restriction and exercise, or control subjects.[75] Participants in the caloric restriction group exhibited more bone density loss at total hip (−2.6%) compared with the caloric restriction/exercise and exercise groups (−1.1%, + 1.5%).[75] In Look-AHEAD, intensive lifestyle participants were at a 39% higher risk of fragility fractures.[73] The POUNDS LOST trial assessed diet-only effects of weight loss in older adults with obesity on bone density,[76] demonstrating weight loss and significant bone density loss at the spine, hip, and femoral neck.[76] Only women demonstrated a significant association between loss of bone density and loss of muscle mass.[76] Recommendations for weight loss in older adults with obesity parallel those to mitigate muscle loss as outlined previously but, in those indicated, consideration for osteoporosis therapy.[59]

Other risks pertain to musculoskeletal injuries and hypoglycemia. The 12-month incidence of injuries related to exercises in older adults was roughly 13.8%.[77] Even in the LIFE study, the risk ratio between the exercise and the education group was no different.[78] Providers also must be mindful of alterations in metabolic variables, particularly hypoglycemia in participants on insulin, because insulin sensitivity improves and reduces its need.

IMPORTANCE OF TREATING OBESITY TO PROMOTE HEALTH AGING

Health care professionals can aid older patients with obesity in losing weight. The goal should to improve physical function and QoL. The quality of care is enhanced in its diagnosis and measurement. Although BMI is helpful, there may be improvements in accuracy by including waist circumference. Health care professionals can counsel patients by promoting multidisciplinary lifestyle interventions. Concurrent dietary, behavioral, and exercise (aerobic/resistance) approaches should be prescribed and recommended because they lead to marked improvements in physical function, metabolic improvements, and can minimizes sarcopenia and osteoporosis. Caloric restriction without a concurrent resistance program may be detrimental; we advise against such an approach. Furthermore, there is a critical need to enhance delivery systems in the primary care setting by[79] changing policy structure and reimbursement mechanisms to permit nonphysicians to deliver intensive behavioral therapy.[18] Monitoring of complications as a result of weight loss–induced metabolic improvements should be considered. We strongly advocate the need for additional community-based, pragmatic, and effectiveness interventions to demedicalize obesity in this population. Clinic-community partnerships are a potential way to help implement an easy, cost-effective method to improve weight management programs.[80] Promising preliminary data[81] show that implementing a community-based weight management program is feasible and acceptable. Treating obesity in older adults can mitigate the significant public health crisis, and reduce health care use and risk of long-term adverse events.

DISCLOSURE

The authors have nothing to disclose.

REFERENCES

1. Ortman JM, Victoria A, Velkoff aHH. An aging nation: the older population in the United States,vCurrent population reports. Washington, DC: US Census Bureau; 2014.

2. Hales CM, Fryar CD, Carroll MD, et al. Differences in obesity prevalence by demographic characteristics and urbanization level among adults in the United States, 2013-2016. JAMA 2018;319(23):2419–29.

3. Villareal DT, Apovian CM, Kushner RF, et al. Obesity in older adults: technical review and position statement of the American Society for Nutrition and NAASO, the Obesity Society. Obes Res 2005;13(11):1849–63.

4. Zizza C, Herring A, Domino M, et al. The effect of weight change on nursing care facility admission in the NHANES I Epidemiologic Followup Survey. J Clin Epidemiol 2003;56(9):906–13.

5. Batsis JA, Mackenzie TA, Barre LK, et al. Sarcopenia, sarcopenic obesity and mortality in older adults. Eur J Clin Nutr 2014;68(9):1001–7.

6. GBD 2015 Obesity Collaborators, Afshin A, Forouzanfar MH, et al. Health effects of overweight and obesity in 195 countries over 25 years. N Engl J Med 2017; 377(1):13–27.

7. Obesity and overweight. 2018. Available at: https://www.who.int/news-room/fact-sheets/detail/obesity-and-overweight. Accessed December 6, 2019.
8. Hales CM, Carroll MD, Fryar CD, et al. Prevalence of obesity among adults and youth: United States, 2015–2016 2017.
9. Befort CA, Nazir N, Perri MG. Prevalence of obesity among adults from rural and urban areas of the United States: findings from NHANES (2005-2008). J Rural Health 2012;28(4):392–7.
10. Fakhouri TH, Ogden CL, Carroll MD, et al. Prevalence of obesity among older adults in the United States, 2007-2010. NCHS Data Brief 2012;(106):1–8.
11. Dinsa GD, Goryakin Y, Fumagalli E, et al. Obesity and socioeconomic status in developing countries: a systematic review. Obes Rev 2012;13(11):1067–79.
12. Conklin AI, Forouhi NG, Suhrcke M, et al. Socioeconomic status, financial hardship and measured obesity in older adults: a cross-sectional study of the EPIC-Norfolk cohort. BMC Public Health 2013;13:1039.
13. Khan SS, Ning H, Wilkins JT, et al. Association of body mass index with lifetime risk of cardiovascular disease and compression of morbidity. JAMA Cardiol 2018;3(4):280–7.
14. Visser M, Pahor M, Tylavsky F, et al. One- and two-year change in body composition as measured by DXA in a population-based cohort of older men and women. J Appl Physiol 2003;94(6):2368–74.
15. Jura M, Kozak LP. Obesity and related consequences to ageing. Age (Dordr) 2016;38(1):23.
16. Hall ME, Clark D 3rd, Jones DW. Fat and cardiometabolic risk: location, location, location. J Clin Hypertens (Greenwich) 2019;21(7):963–5.
17. Batsis JA, Villareal DT. Sarcopenic obesity in older adults: aetiology, epidemiology and treatment strategies. Nat Rev Endocrinol 2018;14(9):513–37.
18. Batsis JA, Gill LE, Masutani RK, et al. Weight loss interventions in older adults with obesity: a systematic review of randomized controlled trials since 2005. J Am Geriatr Soc 2017;65(2):257–68.
19. Kalyani RR, Corriere M, Ferrucci L. Age-related and disease-related muscle loss: the effect of diabetes, obesity, and other diseases. Lancet Diabetes Endocrinol 2014;2(10):819–29.
20. Studenski SA, Peters KW, Alley DE, et al. The FNIH sarcopenia project: rationale, study description, conference recommendations, and final estimates. J Gerontol A Biol Sci Med Sci 2014;69(5):547–58.
21. Park SW, Goodpaster BH, Strotmeyer ES, et al. Accelerated loss of skeletal muscle strength in older adults with type 2 diabetes: the health, aging, and body composition study. Diabetes Care 2007;30(6):1507–12.
22. Goodpaster BH, Park SW, Harris TB, et al. The loss of skeletal muscle strength, mass, and quality in older adults: the health, aging and body composition study. J Gerontol A Biol Sci Med Sci 2006;61(10):1059–64.
23. Ness-Abramof R, Apovian CM. Waist circumference measurement in clinical practice. Nutr Clin Pract 2008;23(4):397–404.
24. Garg A. Regional adiposity and insulin resistance. J Clin Endocrinol Metab 2004;89(9):4206–10.
25. Amarya S, Singh K, Sabharwal M. Health consequences of obesity in the elderly. J Clin Gerontol Geriatr 5(3):63–7.
26. Friedmann JM, Elasy T, Jensen GL. The relationship between body mass index and self-reported functional limitation among older adults: a gender difference. J Am Geriatr Soc 2001;49(4):398–403.

27. Himes CL, Reynolds SL. Effect of obesity on falls, injury, and disability. J Am Geriatr Soc 2012;60(1):124–9.
28. Mitchell RJ, Lord SR, Harvey LA, et al. Associations between obesity and overweight and fall risk, health status and quality of life in older people. Aust N Z J Public Health 2014;38(1):13–8.
29. Ylitalo KR, Karvonen-Gutierrez CA. Body mass index, falls, and injurious falls among U.S. adults: findings from the 2014 Behavioral Risk Factor Surveillance System. Prev Med 2016;91:217–23.
30. Rosenblatt NJ, Grabiner MD. Relationship between obesity and falls by middle-aged and older women. Arch Phys Med Rehabil 2012;93(4):718–22.
31. Scott D, Seibel M, Cumming R, et al. Sarcopenic obesity and its temporal associations with changes in bone mineral density, incident falls, and fractures in older men: the concord health and ageing in men project. J Bone Miner Res 2017; 32(3):575–83.
32. Ozturk ZA, Turkbeyler IH, Abiyev A, et al. Health-related quality of life and fall risk associated with age-related body composition changes; sarcopenia, obesity and sarcopenic obesity. Intern Med J 2018;48(8):973–81.
33. Compston J. Obesity and fractures in postmenopausal women. Curr Opin Rheumatol 2015;27(4):414–9.
34. Fjeldstad C, Fjeldstad AS, Acree LS, et al. The influence of obesity on falls and quality of life. Dyn Med 2008;7:4.
35. You H, Li XL, Jing KZ, et al. Association between body mass index and health-related quality of life among Chinese elderly: evidence from a community-based study. BMC Public Health 2018;18(1):1174.
36. Espeland MA, Luchsinger JA, Baker LD, et al. Effect of a long-term intensive lifestyle intervention on prevalence of cognitive impairment. Neurology 2017;88(21): 2026–35.
37. Horie NC, Serrao VT, Simon SS, et al. Cognitive effects of intentional weight loss in elderly obese individuals with mild cognitive impairment. J Clin Endocrinol Metab 2016;101(3):1104–12.
38. Napoli N, Shah K, Waters DL, et al. Effect of weight loss, exercise, or both on cognition and quality of life in obese older adults. Am J Clin Nutr 2014;100(1): 189–98.
39. Bischof GN, Park DC. Obesity and aging: consequences for cognition, brain structure, and brain function. Psychosom Med 2015;77(6):697–709.
40. Eight-year weight losses with an intensive lifestyle intervention: the look AHEAD study. Obesity (Silver Spring) 2014;22(1):5–13.
41. Musich S, Wang SS, Kraemer S, et al. Purpose in life and positive health outcomes among older adults. Popul Health Manag 2018;21(2):139–47.
42. Harris JA, Castle NG. Obesity and nursing home care in the United States: a systematic review. Gerontologist 2019;59(3):e196–206.
43. Kritchevsky SB, Beavers KM, Miller ME, et al. Intentional weight loss and all-cause mortality: a meta-analysis of randomized clinical trials. PLoS One 2015; 10(3):e0121993.
44. Kalinkovich A, Livshits G. Sarcopenic obesity or obese sarcopenia: a cross talk between age-associated adipose tissue and skeletal muscle inflammation as a main mechanism of the pathogenesis. Ageing Res Rev 2017;35:200–21.
45. Schaap LA, Koster A, Visser M. Adiposity, muscle mass, and muscle strength in relation to functional decline in older persons. Epidemiol Rev 2013;35:51–65.
46. Rolland Y, Lauwers-Cances V, Cristini C, et al. Difficulties with physical function associated with obesity, sarcopenia, and sarcopenic-obesity in community-

dwelling elderly women: the EPIDOS (EPIDemiologie de l'OSteoporose) Study. Am J Clin Nutr 2009;89(6):1895–900.

47. Hirani V, Naganathan V, Blyth F, et al. Longitudinal associations between body composition, sarcopenic obesity and outcomes of frailty, disability, institutionalisation and mortality in community-dwelling older men: the Concord Health and Ageing in Men Project. Age Ageing 2017;46(3):413–20.

48. Batsis JA, Zbehlik AJ, Pidgeon D, et al. Dynapenic obesity and the effect on long-term physical function and quality of life: data from the osteoarthritis initiative. BMC Geriatr 2015;15:118.

49. Valiyeva E, Russell LB, Miller JE, et al. Lifestyle-related risk factors and risk of future nursing home admission. Arch Intern Med 2006;166(9):985–90.

50. Zizza CA, Herring A, Stevens J, et al. Obesity affects nursing-care facility admission among whites but not blacks. Obes Res 2002;10(8):816–23.

51. Lapane KL, Resnik L. Obesity in nursing homes: an escalating problem. J Am Geriatr Soc 2005;53(8):1386–91.

52. Felix HC, Bradway C, Ali MM, et al. Nursing home perspectives on the admission of morbidly obese patients from hospitals to nursing homes. J Appl Gerontol 2016;35(3):286–302.

53. Felix HC, Bradway C, Miller E, et al. Obese nursing home residents: a call to research action. J Am Geriatr Soc 2010;58(6):1196–7.

54. Chang VW, Langa KM, Weir D, et al. The obesity paradox and incident cardiovascular disease: a population-based study. PLoS One 2017;12(12):e0188636.

55. Brown RE, Kuk JL. Consequences of obesity and weight loss: a devil's advocate position. Obes Rev 2015;16(1):77–87.

56. Veronese N, Cereda E, Solmi M, et al. Inverse relationship between body mass index and mortality in older nursing home residents: a meta-analysis of 19,538 elderly subjects. Obes Rev 2015;16(11):1001–15.

57. Flegal KM, Ioannidis JPA. The obesity paradox: a misleading term that should be abandoned. Obesity (Silver Spring) 2018;26(4):629–30.

58. Tobias DK, Hu FB. Does being overweight really reduce mortality? Obesity (Silver Spring) 2013;21(9):1746–9.

59. DiMilia PR, Mittman AC, Batsis JA. Benefit-to-risk balance of weight loss interventions in older adults with obesity. Curr Diab Rep 2019;19(11):114.

60. Batsis JA, Mackenzie TA, Bartels SJ, et al. Diagnostic accuracy of body mass index to identify obesity in older adults: NHANES 1999-2004. Int J Obes (Lond) 2016;40(5):761–7.

61. Haywood C, Sumithran P. Treatment of obesity in older persons: a systematic review. Obes Rev 2019;20(4):588–98.

62. Payne ME, Porter Starr KN, Orenduff M, et al. Quality of life and mental health in older adults with obesity and frailty: associations with a weight loss intervention. J Nutr Health Aging 2018;22(10):1259–65.

63. Fanning J, Walkup MP, Ambrosius WT, et al. Change in health-related quality of life and social cognitive outcomes in obese, older adults in a randomized controlled weight loss trial: does physical activity behavior matter? J Behav Med 2018;41(3):299–308.

64. Villareal DT, Chode S, Parimi N, et al. Weight loss, exercise, or both and physical function in obese older adults. N Engl J Med 2011;364(13):1218–29.

65. Houston DK, Neiberg RH, Miller ME, et al. Physical function following a long-term lifestyle intervention among middle aged and older adults with type 2 diabetes: the look AHEAD study. J Gerontol A Biol Sci Med Sci 2018;73(11):1552–9.

66. Weinheimer EM, Sands LP, Campbell WW. A systematic review of the separate and combined effects of energy restriction and exercise on fat-free mass in middle-aged and older adults: implications for sarcopenic obesity. Nutr Rev 2010;68(7):375–88.

67. Whelton PK, Appel LJ, Espeland MA, et al. Sodium reduction and weight loss in the treatment of hypertension in older persons: a randomized controlled trial of nonpharmacologic interventions in the elderly (TONE). TONE Collaborative Research Group. JAMA 1998;279(11):839–46.

68. Messier SP, Mihalko SL, Legault C, et al. Effects of intensive diet and exercise on knee joint loads, inflammation, and clinical outcomes among overweight and obese adults with knee osteoarthritis: the IDEA randomized clinical trial. JAMA 2013;310(12):1263–73.

69. Bauer J, Biolo G, Cederholm T, et al. Evidence-based recommendations for optimal dietary protein intake in older people: a position paper from the PROT-AGE Study Group. J Am Med Dir Assoc 2013;14(8):542–59.

70. Porter Starr KN, Pieper CF, Orenduff MC, et al. Improved function with enhanced protein intake per meal: a pilot study of weight reduction in frail, obese older adults. J Gerontol A Biol Sci Med Sci 2016;71(10):1369–75.

71. Coker RH, Wolfe RR. Weight loss strategies in the elderly: a clinical conundrum. Obesity (Silver Spring) 2018;26(1):22–8.

72. Zibellini J, Seimon RV, Lee CM, et al. Effect of diet-induced weight loss on muscle strength in adults with overweight or obesity: a systematic review and meta-analysis of clinical trials. Obes Rev 2016;17(8):647–63.

73. Gallagher D, Kelley DE, Thornton J, et al. Changes in skeletal muscle and organ size after a weight-loss intervention in overweight and obese type 2 diabetic patients. Am J Clin Nutr 2017;105(1):78–84.

74. Soltani S, Hunter GR, Kazemi A, et al. The effects of weight loss approaches on bone mineral density in adults: a systematic review and meta-analysis of randomized controlled trials. Osteoporos Int 2016;27(9):2655–71.

75. Shah K, Armamento-Villareal R, Parimi N, et al. Exercise training in obese older adults prevents increase in bone turnover and attenuates decrease in hip bone mineral density induced by weight loss despite decline in bone-active hormones. J Bone Miner Res 2011;26(12):2851–9.

76. Tirosh A, de Souza RJ, Sacks F, et al. Sex differences in the effects of weight loss diets on bone mineral density and body composition: POUNDS LOST trial. J Clin Endocrinol Metab 2015;100(6):2463–71.

77. Little RM, Paterson DH, Humphreys DA, et al. A 12-month incidence of exercise-related injuries in previously sedentary community-dwelling older adults following an exercise intervention. BMJ Open 2013;3(6):e002831.

78. Pahor M, Guralnik JM, Ambrosius WT, et al. Effect of structured physical activity on prevention of major mobility disability in older adults: the LIFE study randomized clinical trial. JAMA 2014;311(23):2387–96.

79. Leblanc ES, O'Connor E, Whitlock EP, et al. Effectiveness of primary care-relevant treatments for obesity in adults: a systematic evidence review for the U.S. Preventive Services Task Force. Ann Intern Med 2011;155(7):434–47.

80. Wilkes AE, John PM, Vable AM, et al. Combating Obesity at Community Health Centers (COACH): a quality improvement collaborative for weight management programs. J Health Care Poor Underserved 2013;24(2 Suppl):47–60.

81. Dodd-Reynolds CJ, Nevens L, Oliver EJ, et al. Prototyping for public health in a local context. BMJ Open 2019;9(10):e029718.

Lifestyle (Medicine) and Healthy Aging

Susan M. Friedman, MD, MPH

KEYWORDS

- Successful aging • Lifestyle medicine • Compression of morbidity • Multimorbidity
- Nutrition • Physical activity

KEY POINTS

- Healthy habits impact longevity and health in old age, leading to a compression of morbidity.
- Together, lifestyle and social circumstances contribute more to the risk of premature mortality than does genetic predisposition.
- Recent population trends have shown an earlier onset of many chronic diseases, with an increase in multimorbidity among older adults. As a result, older adults may experience more disability and a poorer quality of life.
- Lifestyle medicine, the evidence-based practice of helping individuals and families adopt and sustain healthy behaviors that affect health and quality of life, was established to address root causes of disease, and is therefore foundational in trying to reduce the burden of chronic illness.
- Many studies have evaluated the impact of lifestyle medicine "pillars," including nutrition, physical activity, well-being, stress management, and sleep, on outcomes that are important to geriatrics and healthy aging. These outcomes include multimorbidity, functional decline, cognitive health, engagement, frailty, and sarcopenia.

INTRODUCTION

Healthy aging is a process that occurs over the life cycle. Health habits established early and practiced throughout life impact both longevity, the ability to reach old age, and the health with which one experiences older adulthood. The new field of lifestyle medicine (LM) can help to optimize the trajectory of aging, and can promote targets that have been recognized in geriatric medicine as essential to well-being and quality of life. These include preventing or delaying the onset of comorbidity, decline in physical function, decline in cognitive function, and the onset of sarcopenia and frailty. This article reviews the impact of lifestyle on health, describes the field of LM, and reviews literature that outlines the connection between lifestyle and healthy aging.

University of Rochester School of Medicine and Dentistry, 1000 South Avenue, Box 58, Rochester, NY 14620, USA
E-mail address: Susan_Friedman@urmc.rochester.edu

Clin Geriatr Med 36 (2020) 645–653
https://doi.org/10.1016/j.cger.2020.06.007
0749-0690/20/© 2020 Elsevier Inc. All rights reserved.

geriatric.theclinics.com

THE IMPACT OF LIFESTYLE ON HEALTH

Health is the result of a complex interplay between genetic predisposition, socio-behavioral-environmental influences, and access to health care. It has been estimated that behavioral and social circumstances contribute most to premature death[1] (**Fig. 1**). In the United States, behavioral factors strongly impact both longevity and disability-adjusted life-years. A recent article listed dietary risks, tobacco smoking, high body mass index, high blood pressure, high fasting blood glucose, and physical inactivity or low activity as the top risk factors for both of these outcomes.[2]

TRENDS IN HEALTH AND LONGEVITY

From 1990 to 2010, life expectancy increased from 75.2 years to 78.2 years, an increase of 3 years. During that time, healthy life expectancy increased 2.3 years, from 65.8 years to 68.1 years. In other words, life expectancy increased more than healthy life expectancy, so that the number of years spent in poor health also increased, from 9.4 years to 10.1 years.[2]

A central tenet of geriatric medicine has long been the goal of compressing morbidity. In 1980, James Fries[3] suggested that "chronic illness may presumably be postponed by changes in life style," thereby delaying the onset of functional decline. Trends in functional capacity among older adults have varied by cohort over time. The prevalence of activities of daily living (ADL) disability was stable over the 1980s and decreased in the 1990s. During the early part of this century, that improvement continued only for the "oldest old," those 85 and older.[4] Recently, younger cohorts have demonstrated earlier onset of disability, raising the concern that future generations of older adults may experience a higher prevalence of disability, and spend more of their lives disabled and in poor health.

Healthy lifestyle factors have shown different trajectories over time. Rates of smoking have decreased, whereas there has been little change in consumption of fruits and vegetables.[5] Sedentary behavior has increased, particularly among older adults.[6] Obesity has increased significantly.[5]

These changes in lifestyle risk factors, in addition to increases in life expectancy, have contributed to the rising prevalence of chronic disease and multimorbidity.

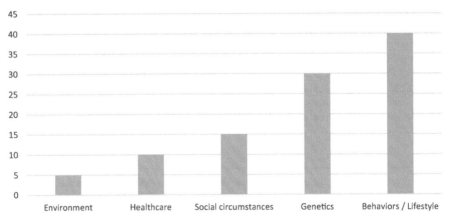

Fig. 1. Contributors to premature mortality. (*Data from* McGinnis JM, Williams-Russo P, Knickman JR. The case for more active policy attention to health promotion. Health Aff (Millwood) 2002;21:78-93.)

Data from the Health and Retirement Study showed an increase in the prevalence of hypertension, diabetes, cancer, chronic obstructive pulmonary disease, and arthritis among older adults. The prevalence of 4 or more chronic diseases increased from 11.6% to 17.4% during the decade from 1998 to 2008. During that same interval, the proportion of older adults with no chronic illness decreased from 13.1% to 7.8%.[7] In other words, multimorbidity is on the rise, and the likelihood of living to old age without chronic illness is declining.

Since 2014, life expectancy itself has decreased each year, driven by an increase in mortality rates in individuals aged 25 to 64 in all racial groups.[8] The greatest increases have resulted from the "diseases of despair" (drug overdoses and suicide), and organ system diseases. This reduces the likelihood that an individual will reach old age at all, whether healthy or unhealthy.

WHAT IS LIFESTYLE MEDICINE?

Paul Batalden, of the Institute for Healthcare Improvement, has been quoted as saying "Every system is perfectly designed to get the results it gets." Along with the rise in chronic disease, we are seeing tremendous growth in health expenditures. Health care costs more than doubled from 2000 to 2017, going from $1.4 trillion to $3.5 trillion.[9]

In response, the American College of Lifestyle Medicine was founded in 2004, with a mission of advancing evidence-based LM to prevent, treat, and reverse chronic disease. LM has been defined as "the evidence-based practice of helping individuals and families adopt and sustain healthy behaviors that affect health and quality of life."[10] By addressing root causes of chronic disease, LM seeks to go beyond the management of an ever-increasing burden of chronic disease, focusing on preventing, delaying, and at times reversing its onset and progression.

By its nature, LM is collaborative; it requires active participation by the patients involved. Patients are therefore both engaged and empowered to promote the outcome of good health.

In 2015, the American Board of Lifestyle Medicine was established, and the first Boards in LM were administered in 2017. Recommendations for LM competencies included assessment and management of the "pillars" of the field, including tobacco, alcohol, diet, physical activity, weight, stress, sleep, and emotional well-being[11] (**Box 1**).

WHAT IS HEALTHY AGING?

Healthy aging is defined in much greater detail in Louise Aronson's article, "Healthy Aging Across the Stages of Old Age," in this issue but we briefly review the definition

---

Box 1
Pillars of lifestyle medicine

- Tobacco
- Alcohol and other substances
- Nutrition
- Physical activity
- Weight
- Stress
- Sleep
- Emotional well-being

and principles here. The World Health Organization has defined active and healthy aging as "the process of optimizing opportunities for health, participation, and security in order to enhance quality of life as people age." This definition acknowledges that healthy aging is a product of an environment and of systems that help to promote health and vitality for all. Healthy aging is a multidimensional concept that includes physical, mental, social, economic, cultural, spiritual, and civic components.

Perhaps the most well-known framework for describing successful aging was put forward by Rowe and Kahn in 1998[12] (**Box 2**) This model includes 3 components: avoiding disease, maintaining high cognitive and physical function, and remaining engaged with life. The intersection of these 3 realms represents an optimal situation, which they termed "healthy aging." However, most people will develop 1 or more chronic diseases in their lifetime. The proportion of older adults without any chronic illness is less than 8%.[7] When older adults are surveyed about their goals, and how they envision healthy aging, they tend to focus more on engagement, maintaining independence, and belonging to a community.[13] Through adaptation and compensation, there is a recognition that a life of meaning, purpose, and connectedness is still feasible in the setting of chronic illness and functional decline.

Box 2
Components of successful aging: Rowe and Kahn model

- Avoiding disease
- Maintaining cognitive and physical function
- Preserving engagement

EVIDENCE THAT LIFESTYLE CONTRIBUTES TO HEALTHY AGING

Although much work has yet to be done to fully understand the connections between lifestyle and healthy aging (**Fig. 2**), there is a growing body of literature that addresses these connections. Several of these lifestyle (eg, nutrition, physical activity, stress) and geriatric (eg, multimorbidity, cognition, physical function, engagement, frailty) domains are addressed in detail in other articles in this issue, but we review literature that supports these connections.

LIFESTYLE AND CHRONIC DISEASE

Several studies have demonstrated an association of lifestyle with lower risk of developing chronic illness. In the European Prospective Investigation into Cancer and Nutrition–Potsdam Study, 23,000 subjects who were 35 to 65 at baseline were followed for 8 years to determine risk for developing chronic disease. Four lifestyle factors were assessed at baseline: never having smoked; having a body mass index less than 30; physical activity ≥ 3.5 hours per week; and high intake of fruits, vegetables, and whole grains, with low intake of meat. Subjects who had all 4 factors at baseline had a 78% lower risk of developing chronic disease at follow-up, with a 93% lower risk of developing diabetes, 81% lower risk of having a myocardial infarction, 50% lower risk of stroke, and 36% lower risk of being diagnosed with cancer.[14]

Several studies have demonstrated that therapeutic lifestyle changes can reverse disease that has already been established. In the 1-year Lifestyle Heart Trial, 48 subjects with established coronary artery disease were randomized to a multidimensional

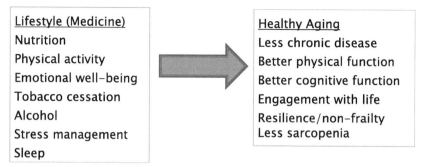

Fig. 2. Connections between LM and healthy aging.

lifestyle intervention versus usual care. Average age was 56, with a range from 35 to 75. The intervention consisted of a very low-fat (10% of calories from fat) vegetarian diet, smoking cessation, stress management (stretching, breathing, meditation, progressive relaxation, and imagery for an hour per day), moderate exercise, and twice weekly support sessions facilitated by a psychologist. Subjects underwent cardiac catheterization at baseline and 1 year later. Eighty-two percent of the intervention group had regression of disease. The intervention group had 91% fewer angina episodes, whereas the control group had 165% more than baseline. Total cholesterol fell by 24%, and low-density lipoprotein fell by 37%. There was a strong dose-response relationship, so that subjects who had the highest adherence had the most improvement.[15]

LIFESTYLE AND DISABILITY

Lester Breslow was one of the first investigators to look at connections between lifestyle and health. In the Alameda County study, he followed almost 7000 subjects, looking at 7 healthy habits: avoiding smoking, drinking in moderation, sleeping 7 or 8 hours per night, exercising at least moderately, eating regular meals, maintaining a moderate weight, and eating breakfast. Those with 6 or more healthy habits lived 11 years longer than those with 3 or fewer, and were less likely to become disabled. Of those with 4 or more healthy habits at baseline, 12.2% were likely to be disabled 10 years after the study began. Those with 2 or 3 had a 14.1% likelihood, and those with 0 to 1 had an 18.7% likelihood of being disabled.[16] Other studies have confirmed the protective effect of healthy lifestyle, with those engaged in healthy behaviors having up to 75% lower likelihood of becoming disabled compared with those who did not engage in healthy behaviors.[17]

Among older adults, a community-based cohort study of 5248 men and women aged 65 and older from 4 communities evaluated duration of life free of difficulties with ADLs, comparing healthy and unhealthy lifestyles. They looked at 7 components (**Table 1**). For each group (White and Black women and men), , individuals who had a healthy lifestyle had a higher active life expectancy than the total life expectancy for those who had an unhealthy lifestyle. This demonstrates not only an increase in longevity, but a compression of morbidity, for those with a healthy lifestyle.[18]

LIFESTYLE AND COGNITIVE DECLINE

A great deal of work has been done recently to evaluate the potential impact of lifestyle on preserving cognition and preventing dementia. This is discussed fully in

Table 1 Lifestyle components predicting preservation of function		
Lifestyle Component	Healthy	Unhealthy
Smoking	Never	Current
Alcohol	1–7 drinks per wk	14+ drinks per wk
Body mass index	18–24.9	30+
Exercise	2300 kcal leisure activity per wk	375 kcal leisure activity per wk
Walking	48 blocks per wk	6 blocks per wk
Social network	Top quartile	Bottom quartile
Social support	Top quartile	Bottom quartile

Maryjo L. Cleveland's article, "Preserving Cognition, Preventing Dementia," elsewhere in this issue, but will be addressed briefly here. The Alzheimer's Association recently reviewed several modifiable risk factors for cognitive decline, and separately for dementia. They found sufficiently strong evidence that regular physical activity and management of cardiovascular risk factors (diabetes, obesity, smoking and hypertension) reduce risk of cognitive decline, and may reduce risk of dementia. Healthy diet and lifelong learning/cognitive training may also reduce the risk of cognitive decline.[19]

The FINGER trial, which is currently being replicated in multiple sites in the United States, enrolled 1260 at-risk individuals aged 60 to 77 with CAIDE Dementia Risk Score of 6 or more and cognitive performance at the mean or slightly low for expected age (eg, Mini Mental State Examination 20–26) in a 2-year randomized controlled trial. The multidimensional intervention included nutritional guidance, physical exercise, cognitive training and social activity, and intensive monitoring and management of metabolic and vascular risk factors. At 2 years, controls had an odds ratio of 1.31 ($P = .04$) for cognitive decline. Impact was greatest on executive functioning (83% higher than controls) and processing speed (150% higher than controls).[20,21]

In a prospective cohort study of 1880 community-dwelling older adults, individuals who exercised approximately 2.5 hours per week had a hazard ratio of 0.67 of developing Alzheimer dementia. Those with a high adherence to a Mediterranean-type diet had a risk that was 40% lower than those who did not. Absolute risk reduction for high adherence to diet and exercise was 12% (from 21% to 9%), for a number needed to treat of 8.[22]

LIFESTYLE AND ENGAGEMENT

Remaining engaged is 1 of the 3 components of successful aging in the model proposed by Rowe and Kahn.[12] Engagement is a multifaceted concept that includes interpersonal relationships; social participation; leisure, social, and fitness activities; and productive activities. It is the least well studied component of the successful aging model, although it is the focus of what many older adults identify as the key component of healthy or successful aging. It is also at the top of a hierarchy, such that, when chronic disease is absent, it is easier to maintain physical and cognitive function, and when function is preserved, it is easier to remain engaged.[23] On the other hand, social engagement may support preservation of function,[24] as maintaining a sense of meaning, purpose, and connectedness fosters physical activity.

Involvement in physical activity and fitness activities leads to heightened social engagement. Even in very frail older adults, participation in fitness training has been shown to result in increased spontaneous activity,[25] which may in turn reduce barriers to socialization. In one study, older adults who were physically inactive were approximately 40% more likely to report being socially disengaged.[26]

The World Health Organization describes healthy aging as "the process of optimizing opportunities for health, participation and security in order to enhance quality of life as people age." It has been recognized that environment is key in both promoting and removing barriers to engagement. Projects such as the AARP Age-Friendly Communities, and Blue Zones replications, have demonstrated that developing the built environment and programs that acknowledge the needs of older adults along a spectrum of function, can help to foster engagement.[27]

LIFESTYLE, SARCOPENIA, AND FRAILTY

Sarcopenia is the presence of low muscle mass with low strength and/or physical performance, seen with aging. It puts older adults at risk of frailty, falls, and functional decline. Prevalence has been estimated to be up to 15% in those older than 65, and up to 50% in those older than 80. Knee and elbow strength decline at a rate of 1% to 4% per year in older adults, with men having more rapid declines than women, and the loss of muscle strength outpacing the loss of muscle mass.[28]

Several different lifestyle components reduce the risk of sarcopenia, which results from decreased muscle protein synthesis, increased muscle protein degradation, and decreased muscle function and quality.[29] Sedentary lifestyle is a major risk factor for sarcopenia, and, conversely, exercise is an important strategy in preventing and treating it. Both aerobic activity and resistance training are important for maintaining muscle mass and strength, and general physical activity may help to prevent sarcopenia.[28,29] There is no threshold for association, so that even people with very low levels of activity can benefit from small increases in aerobic exercise and resistance training. Progressive resistance training programs should include 8 to 12 repetitions per muscle group of 60% to 80% of the 1-repetition maximum, and should be done 3 times weekly to combat sarcopenia.

Longitudinal studies have suggested that dietary protein intake is important in protecting against sarcopenia. The protein recommended dietary allowance for younger adults is 0.8 g/kg per day, and there is evidence that older adults may need 1.1 g/kg per day.[29] Vitamin D is important in maintaining muscle strength through maintaining the function of type II fibers. There is growing literature to suggest that diets high in fruits, vegetables, and carotenoids, which are protective against oxidative stress, may also protect against developing sarcopenia. A recent meta-analysis of the Mediterranean diet and frailty in older adults showed that the more adherent people were to a Mediterranean diet, which is high in vegetables, legumes, fruit and nuts, and low in saturated fat and red and processed meat, the lower their risk of developing frailty. Subjects with a Mediterranean diet score of 6 to 9 had more than a 50% relative risk reduction of developing frailty, compared with those with a diet score of 3 or less.[30]

Chronic alcohol misuse can lead to myopathy characterized by atrophy of type II fibers, and affects approximately 50% of alcohol misusers. It is reversible with abstinence. Smoking also increases the risk of sarcopenia, through impairing both muscle protein synthesis and maintenance.

SUMMARY

Lifestyle influences both longevity and health in old age. This, in turn, leads to a compression of morbidity, which has long been a goal of geriatric medicine. Recently, life expectancy has decreased in the United States among young and middle-aged adults, and people are experiencing earlier onset of disease and more chronic comorbidities. LM, the evidence-based practice of helping individuals and families develop and maintain healthy behaviors, treats the root causes of chronic disease. LM evaluates and treats nutrition, physical activity, well-being, stress management, substance use, connectedness, and sleep, to prevent, arrest, and reverse chronic illness. In so doing, LM can lead to outcomes that have been important to geriatrics, such as reducing multimorbidity, preventing or delaying functional and cognitive decline, reducing frailty, and maintaining engagement, which all contribute to health in old age.

DISCLOSURE

The author has nothing to disclose.

REFERENCES

1. Schroeder SA. Shattuck Lecture. We can do better–improving the health of the American people. N Engl J Med 2007;357(12):1221–8.
2. Murray CJ, Atkinson C, Bhalla K, et al. The state of US health, 1990-2010: burden of diseases, injuries, and risk factors. JAMA 2013;310(6):591–608.
3. Fries JF. Aging, natural death, and the compression of morbidity. N Engl J Med 1980;303(3):130–5.
4. Crimmins EM. Lifespan and healthspan: past, present, and promise. Gerontologist 2015;55(6):901–11.
5. Troost JP, Rafferty AP, Luo Z, et al. Temporal and regional trends in the prevalence of healthy lifestyle characteristics: United States, 1994-2007. Am J Public Health 2012;102(7):1392–8.
6. Ladabaum U, Mannalithara A, Myer PA, et al. Obesity, abdominal obesity, physical activity, and caloric intake in US adults: 1988 to 2010. Am J Med 2014;127(8): 717–727 e712.
7. Hung WW, Ross JS, Boockvar KS, et al. Recent trends in chronic disease, impairment and disability among older adults in the United States. BMC Geriatr 2011; 11:47.
8. Woolf SH, Schoomaker H. Life expectancy and mortality rates in the United States, 1959-2017. JAMA 2019;322(20):1996–2016.
9. Kamal R, Cox C. How has US spending on healthcare changed over time? 2018 2019. Available at: https://www.healthsystemtracker.org/chart-collection/u-s-spending-healthcare-changed-time/#item-health-services-spending-growth-slowed-a-bit-in-recent-quarters_2018. Accessed November 21, 2019.
10. Physician competencies for prescribing lifestyle medicine. 2019. Available at: https://www.lifestylemedicine.org/ACLM/About/What_is_Lifestyle_Medicine_/Core_Competencies.aspx. Accessed December 9, 2019.
11. Lianov L, Johnson M. Physician competencies for prescribing lifestyle medicine. JAMA 2010;304(2):202–3.
12. Rowe JW, Kahn RL. Successful aging. New York.: Pantheon Books; 1998.
13. Cosco TD, Prina AM, Perales J, et al. Lay perspectives of successful ageing: a systematic review and meta-ethnography. BMJ Open 2013;3(6).
14. Ford ES, Bergmann MM, Kroger J, et al. Healthy living is the best revenge: findings from the European Prospective Investigation into Cancer and Nutrition-Potsdam study. Arch Intern Med 2009;169(15):1355–62.
15. Ornish D, Brown SE, Scherwitz LW, et al. Can lifestyle changes reverse coronary heart disease? The Lifestyle Heart Trial. Lancet 1990;336(8708):129–33.

16. Belloc NB, Breslow L. Relationship of physical health status and health practices. Prev Med 1972;1(3):409–21.
17. Liao W, Li C, Lin YC, et al. Healthy behaviors and onset of functional disability in older adults: results of a national longitudinal study. J Am Geriatr Soc 2011;59(2): 200–6.
18. Jacob ME, Yee LM, Diehr PH, et al. Can a healthy lifestyle compress the disabled period in older adults? J Am Geriatr Soc 2016;64(10):1952–61.
19. Baumgart M, Snyder HM, Carrillo MC, et al. Summary of the evidence on modifiable risk factors for cognitive decline and dementia: a population-based perspective. Alzheimers Dement 2015;11(6):718–26.
20. Ngandu T, Lehtisalo J, Solomon A, et al. A 2 year multidomain intervention of diet, exercise, cognitive training, and vascular risk monitoring versus control to prevent cognitive decline in at-risk elderly people (FINGER): a randomised controlled trial. Lancet 2015;385(9984):2255–63.
21. Kivipelto M, Solomon A, Ahtiluoto S, et al. The Finnish geriatric intervention study to prevent cognitive impairment and disability (FINGER): study design and progress. Alzheimers Dement 2013;9(6):657–65.
22. Scarmeas N, Luchsinger JA, Schupf N, et al. Physical activity, diet, and risk of Alzheimer disease. JAMA 2009;302(6):627–37.
23. Liffiton JA, Horton S, Baker J, et al. Successful aging: how does physical activity influence engagement with life? Eur Rev Aging Phys Act 2012;9:103–8.
24. Menec VH. The relation between everyday activities and successful aging: a 6-year longitudinal study. J Gerontol B Psychol Sci Soc Sci 2003;58(2):S74–82.
25. Fiatarone MA, O'Neill EF, Ryan ND, et al. Exercise training and nutritional supplementation for physical frailty in very elderly people. N Engl J Med 1994;330(25): 1769–75.
26. Meisner BA, Dogra S, Logan AJ, et al. Do or decline? Comparing the effects of physical inactivity on biopsychosocial components of successful aging. J Health Psychol 2010;15(5):688–96.
27. Friedman SM, Mulhausen P, Cleveland ML, et al. American Geriatrics Society White Paper on Healthy Aging. J Am Geriatr Soc 2019. Available at: https://geriatricscareonline.org/toc/american-geriatrics-society-white-paper-on-healthy-aging/CL025.
28. Scott D, Blizzard L, Fell J, et al. The epidemiology of sarcopenia in community living older adults: what role does lifestyle play? J Cachexia Sarcopenia Muscle 2011;2(3):125–34.
29. Rom O, Kaisari S, Aizenbud D, et al. Lifestyle and sarcopenia-etiology, prevention, and treatment. Rambam Maimonides Med J 2012;3(4):e0024.
30. Kojima G, Avgerinou C, Iliffe S, et al. Adherence to Mediterranean diet reduces incident frailty risk: systematic review and meta-analysis. J Am Geriatr Soc 2018;66(4):783–8.

Nutrition and Healthy Aging

Marissa Black, MD, MPH[a,b,c],*, Megan Bowman, MS, RDN[d,e,1]

KEYWORDS

- Older adults • Nutrition • Healthy aging • Diet • Dietary pattern

KEY POINTS

- The predictors of an individual's diet are complex and influenced by multiple socioeconomic, environmental, and behavioral domains.
- Dietary behavior change in late life requires an in-depth understanding of internal and external factors influencing the individual.
- Diet plays a major role in prevention and management of chronic diseases.
- A healthy dietary pattern for older adults is nutrient dense and rich in unprocessed fruit, vegetables, and whole grains.

If we could give every individual the right amount of nourishment and exercise, not too little and not too much, we will have found the safest way to health.
—*Hippocrates (400 BC)*

NUTRITION AND AGING

Nutrition is a key determinant of health throughout the lifecycle, and attention to everyday food behaviors, diet, and lifestyle is a cornerstone of good clinical care. Healthy aging, maintenance of function, immunity, and healing are supported by a high-quality diet that meets micronutrient (vitamin C, A, D, E, and K; zinc; folate; calcium; iron; and B vitamins) and macronutrient (protein, carbohydrate, and fat) requirements.[1–7] Healthy diet with the appropriate balance of nutrients can prevent or delay the development and complications of not only common chronic diseases such as diabetes, high blood pressure, heart disease, and cancer but also diseases,

[a] EvergreenHealth Geriatric Care, 1521 NE 128th Street #100, Kirkland, WA 98034, USA; [b] Division of Gerontology and Geriatric Medicine, Department of Medicine, University of Washington, 1959 NE Pacific, Seattle, WA 98195, USA; [c] Veteran Affairs, GRECC Puget Sound, 1660 South Columbian Way, Mail-stop S-182, Seattle, WA 98118, USA; [d] Veteran Affairs Salt Lake City Health Care System, 500 Foothill Drive, Mail Code 120, Lake City, UT 84148, USA; [e] Department of Exercise Science, Salt Lake Community College, 4600 Redwood Road, Salt Lake City, UT 84123, USA
[1] Present Address: Veteran Affairs Salt Lake City Health Care System, 500 Foothill Drive, Mail Code 120, Lake City, UT 84148.
* Corresponding author: EvergreenHealth Geriatric Care, 1521 NE 128th Street #100, Kirkland, WA 98034.
E-mail address: blackmarissa@gmail.com

Clin Geriatr Med 36 (2020) 655–669
https://doi.org/10.1016/j.cger.2020.06.008
0749-0690/20/© 2020 Elsevier Inc. All rights reserved.

conditions, and outcomes traditionally associated with aging: osteomalacia, osteoporosis, muscle weakness, frailty, falls, pressure sores, hip fractures, hospitalizations, rehospitalizations, and ultimately premature mortality.[5,7,8]

Multiple intrinsic and extrinsic factors influence how older adults acquire, prepare, and consume food: normal and disabling physiologic changes, chronic disease and associated medications, access to food, relationship to food, socioeconomic status, and social isolation (**Fig. 1, Table 1**).[9] These factors contribute to making older adults less likely to meet recommended daily values of nutrients and can contribute to malnutrition.[10–12] Malnutrition in the aging population is associated with declines in functionality (ie, ability to perform activities of daily living) and cognition, thereby further exacerbating problems with intake. The net impact is poor quality of life. Some of these factors are modifiable and good targets for interventions. A wide range of culturally sensitive dietary recommendations and medical nutrition therapy can decrease chronic disease risk and/or slow disease progression.[13] To maintain older adult independence, well-being, and ensure successful aging, tailored care along with national, state, and local strategies to coordinate food and nutrition services is essential.[13] Geriatric providers, as public health advocates and a part of the interdisciplinary care team, can encourage clinical encounters and programming that supports older adults to meet their nutrient requirements.

FRAMEWORK AND OVERVIEW OF DIETARY AND NUTRIENT NEEDS OF OLDER ADULTS

The dietary needs of older adults are multidimensional and the only one component of healthy aging. Because rates of disability, physiologic, and functional impairment are prevalent due to both the normal aging process and underlying disease, older adults are predisposed to nutritional disorders of both underconsumption (eg, B-12 or iron deficiency) and overconsumption (eg, diabetes type II).

BODY COMPOSITION

Normal healthy aging is associated with significant changes in body composition and organ function. The body's water content, bone mass, and lean mass all decrease,

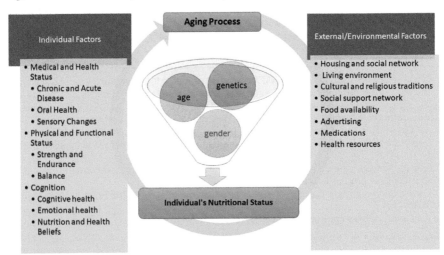

Fig. 1. Contributing Factors to Nutritional Status

Table 1
Intrinsic and extrinsic factors influencing nutritional status and aging process

Extrinsic	
Environmental	Lack of access to healthy food, advertising/media, geopolitics
Medications	Antidepressants, antipsychotics, opioids, laxatives, diabetes medications, steroids, use of more than 4 medications
Social	Death of a spouse, change in housing, isolation from family and friends
Functional	Inability to shop and/or prepare food; inability to feed self; lack of balance, strength, and endurance
Intrinsic	
Physiologic	
Ocular	Visual loss due to aging (reduced acuity, accommodation, depth perception), macular degeneration, glaucoma, cataracts, retinopathy
Neurologic	Parkinson disease, dementia, peripheral neuropathy, gait deficits
Gastrointestinal	Oral problems such as tooth loss, nausea/vomiting, gastrointestinal dysfunction, for example, malabsorption, atrophic gastritis, dysphagia, loss of taste and smell
Cardiovascular/ Pulmonary	Dyspnea
Urologic	Incontinence
Endocrine	Insulin resistance, diabetes type 2, altered or increased metabolic demands/cachexia
Musculoskeletal	Osteoarthritis, pain, weakness
Psychological/ Cognitive	Depression or anxiety, confusion/cognitive decline, loneliness

whereas fat mass generally increases. This increase in fat mass often includes increased abdominal fat stores. Loss of skeletal muscle, as well as gains in total body fat and visceral fat content continue into old age.[14] Consequently, well-standardized nutrient requirements for adults cannot be generalized to older adults.

Body mass index (BMI) is the most practical and the universal anthropometric measurement used for assessing weight status (BMI = weight in kg/height in m^2). BMI does not reflect common body composition changes, nor does it account for height loss that comes with age. Therefore, normal BMI parameters for individuals aged 65 years and older should be between 23 and 30.[15] In addition to BMI, consider ideal body weight, percentage of ideal body weight, usual body weight, and unintended weight loss as measures of weight and nutritional status.

PHYSIOLOGIC CHANGES

Organ function—skin, renal, cardiac, liver, brain—declines at variable rates but can affect nutritional assessment and interventions.

Food consumption requires vision, olfaction, and taste. Rates of visual and smell impairment increase with age and may affect up to 50% of older adults.[16–19] Poor oral health—edentulism and dental problems, xerostomia, and slowed swallowing—affects more than two-thirds of older adults.[20–22] These factors contribute to gustatory dysfunction and less diverse meal composition.[23] Age affects gut motility, saliva production, digestive enzymes (eg, pepsin), pancreatic function, and mucosal immune response of the gut, as well as the postprandial response.[24] Normal aging is associated with a reduction of fluid intake due to diminished thirst sensation, impaired response to serum osmolality, anxiety about toileting, kidneys' reduced ability to concentrate the urine, adverse medication affects, and age-related changes in the hypothalamic region of the brain.

PSYCHOLOGICAL AND SOCIAL FACTORS

Common psychological factors in older adults that are often accompanied by loss of appetite or change in food consumption are depression, dementia or cognitive impairment, or other mood disorders.[25] Social factors such as loneliness, social isolation, poverty, recent change in housing, or death of a partner, all negatively affect eating habits.[26,27] Additional factors that contribute are cultural beliefs, income, education, and functional impairment in mobility and dexterity, which render the complex tasks of cooking and shopping more difficult.[28]

COMORBIDITY AND POLYPHARMACY

Older adults have complex health profiles; more than two-thirds of adults older than 65 years have 2 or more chronic conditions. Older adults are more likely to have cognitive impairment and take multiple medications.[29,30] Polypharmacy, commonly defined as taking greater than 5 medications, is frequent in older adults.[31] Polypharmacy may affect nutritional status and is associated with reduced intake of fiber, fat soluble, and B vitamins and minerals, and increased intake of cholesterol, glucose, and sodium (**Box 1**).[32] Therefore, limiting the number of prescriptions or deprescribing may help with dietary intake.

INTAKE

Intakes tend to decline with advancing age. Unfortunately, diet quality of an average American older than 65 years is poor. The Healthy Eating Index 2010, a measure of diet quality, indicated that the average diet for older adults is lowest for whole grains, greens and beans, and dairy.[33]

ENERGY

Resting energy expenditure is the principle contributor to total energy expenditure.

Box 1
Medications interfering with nutrition
Antipsychotics
Sedative/Hypnotics
Antidepressants
Diabetes drugs
Opiates
Laxatives
Diuretics
Steroids

Total and resting energy requirements decrease with age at about a rate of 100 to 150 kcal/d per decade.[34,35] The decline in energy requirement is multifactorial; however, it is mostly attributable to decreased physical activity. Physical inactivity leads to loss of lean mass, which declines by about 15% between the third and eighth decade of life, leading to lower basal metabolic rate and therefore less demand for energy (calories). The Harris Benedict, or similar equations, can be used to estimate energy needs. Although energy needs decline with age, individuals often do not reduce energy intake leading to increased body fat content.[36,37]

Despite older adults' lower energy requirements, vitamin and mineral needs remain constant or increase. Thus, older adults require a nutrient-dense diet that does not exceed energy requirements.[38,39]

MACRONUTRIENTS: WHAT IS THE OPTIMAL ENERGY SOURCE?

A broad range of carbohydrate-protein-fat ratios can achieve good health and low chronic disease. The focus should be on nutrient quality.[13,40] No single diet is a panacea, but higher quality diets are associated with better quality of life.[41]

FAT

The Food and Nutrition Board recommends a balanced diet of 20% to 35% energy as fat, particularly high in monosaturated and polyunsaturated fats (linoleic acid [n-6] [g/d]: 5% to 10% and alpha-linolenic Acid [n-3] [g/d]: 0.6%–1.2%), reduced intake of dietary cholesterol and saturated fat, and no transfatty acids. In practical terms, direct patients to healthy fats by recommending liquid vegetable oils, eating omega-3–rich foods daily (nuts, seeds, small fish), and limiting red meat and dairy.[38,40,42]

CARBOHYDRATES

Carbohydrates are an important energy source and should constitute 45% to 65% of total energy intake. Fiber-rich, complex carbohydrates, particularly unrefined whole grains, are packed with B vitamins, vitamin E, phytochemicals, and healthy fats.[43,44]

FIBER

Daily fiber recommendations for those aged 60 years or older is at least 30 g for men and 21 g for women or at minimum 14 g fiber per 1000 kcal. Fiber improves gastric motility, glycemic control, and reduces cholesterol; increased fiber intake has been associated with decreased all-cause mortality, decreased incidence of diabetes type 2, coronary artery disease, and colorectal cancer.[44] Fiber rich foods—fruit, vegetables, and whole grains—often have higher nutrient composition and lead to increased satiety. When increasing the fiber content in the diet of an older adult, fluid requirements must also be assessed.

PROTEIN

Consumption of high-quality protein may be challenging for adults as it is often expensive, and older adults may have reduced appetite and physical and environmental limitations.

Protein requirements are recommended at 0.8 g/kg/d, approximately 10% to 35% of total energy, but with stress, hypermetabolic state, increased exercise, and injury, protein requirements are typically estimated closer to 1.5 g/kg/d and up to 2 g/kg/d. Studies show mixed results, but overall short-term nitrogen balance studies suggest

Table 2
Nutrients of concern in older adults

Nutrient	Confirmed Benefits	Source	Quantity[c]
Vitamin D[a,b]	Delay and prevention of progression of osteoporosis	Difficult to obtain from food alone; fish liver oils, flesh of fatty fish, egg yolk, fortified dairy, fortified cereals	51–70y: 600 IU/d 71y: 800 IU/d
Calcium	Delay and prevention of progression of osteoporosis	Dairy, calcium-set tofu, Chinese cabbage, kale, broccoli, fortified foods and beverages	Men 51–70 y: 1000 mg/d ≥71 y: 1200 mg/d Women ≥51 y: 1200 mg/d
Vitamin B12[d]	Prevention of macrocytic anemia, impaired sensory and motor function, and neurocognitive impairment	Fortified cereals, meat, fish, poultry	≥51 y: 2.4 µg/d
Folic acid[e]	Prevention of mental status decline	Enriched cereal grains, beans, peas and lentils, dark leafy vegetables, enriched whole grains, fortified ready-to-eat cereals	≥51 y: 400 µg/d
Iron	Component of hemoglobin and several enzymes, immune system functioning	Nonheme plant sources: fruits, vegetables, fortified breads, and cereals; heme animal sources: meat, poultry	≥51 y: 8 mg/d

[a] Cholecalciferol. 1 µg cholecalciferol = 40 IU vitamin D.

[b] In the absence of adequate exposure to sunlight.

[c] Dietary reference intakes (DRIs): recommended dietary allowances and adequate intakes, vitamins and elements. DRIs is a set of reference values used to plan and assess nutrient intakes of healthy people.

[d] Because 10% to 30% of older adults may malabsorb food-bound B12, it is advisable that those older than 50 years meet their recommended dietary allowances mainly by consuming food fortified with B12 or a supplement containing B12.

[e] As dietary folate equivalents (DFE). 1 DFE = 1 µg food folate = 0.6 µg of folic acid from fortified food or as a supplement consumed with food = 0.5 µg of a supplement taken on an empty stomach.

that the requirement for dietary protein is not different between apparently healthy younger and older adults. In general, it is recommended that older adults obtain at least 1.2 g/kg/d distributed between meals.[11]

FLUID

Dehydration is the most common fluid or electrolyte disturbance in older adults. Generally, older adults require 30 mL/kg/d or 1 mL/kcal ingested (2–4 L) fluids per day. Fluid needs increase with fever, infection, or with diuretic or laxative therapy. Recommended fluids include water, coffee, tea, and other unsweetened beverages.

SALT

Decreased sodium intake will most likely reduce blood pressure and decrease cardiovascular disease morbidity and mortality.[45]

Approximately 77% of dietary sodium intake is from processed foods, and less than 10% is added at the table or during cooking. Recommended intake of salt is approximately 1.5 g/d, whereas average intake is 5.6 g/d.[2,46]

MICRONUTRIENTS

A healthy diet, rich in vitamins and minerals, is vital to optimal functioning. Bioavailability, absorption, and storage of vitamins and minerals is affected by age, gender, genetics, nutritional status, dietary intake, fiber content of the diet, prescription drugs, and alcohol usage. Foods are the safest, most effective, and enjoyable source of vitamins and minerals. Vitamin and mineral supplementation should only be suggested with poor dietary intake or when a diet is known to be deficient, and in some cases, individual supplementation may be warranted (**Table 2**).

DIETARY ASSESSMENT

A complete geriatric assessment incorporates dietary history. A dietary history incorporates medical history, review of systems, surgical history, medications, allergies, sociocultural and instrumental activities of daily living, socioeconomic history, and food insecurity screening. Specific tactics can be used to obtain a dietary intake

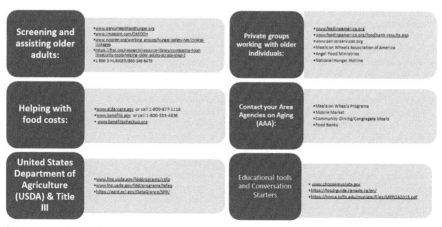

Fig. 2. Resources guide.

history, including documenting usual intake, administering a 24-hour recall or food frequency questionnaire, or obtaining a 3-day food record.[47,48]

When counseling patients on healthy eating, use practical tools, motivational interviewing, and problem solve together (**Fig. 2, Table 3**). In addition, use team-based care and consult your local registered dietitian nutritionist for assistance in patients with heart disease, certain cancers, cerebrovascular disease, diabetes mellitus, renal disease, obesity, or those interested in specialized diets.

FOOD INSECURITY AND HEALTH: SCREEN, INTERVENE, AND ADVOCATE FOR CHANGE

Food insecurity is the lack of consistent access to enough food for an active, healthy life (United States Department of Agriculture). Food insecurity among older adults can have particularly deleterious effects including declines in health and cognitive function, increases in chronic disease, and diminished ability to maintain independence.[49]

It is well-known that food security promotes health, yet in 2017, 50 million (~8%) adults aged 65 years and older experience food insecurity, and by 2030, the number is expected to increase to 73 million. Food insecure adults are more likely to be in poor health and suffer multiple comorbidities.[50,51] In the primary care setting, we can screen for food insecurity, intervene by educating peers about connections between food insecurity and poor health, establish working relationships with community partners to assist patients, as well as engage with food policy councils to add expert health professional perspectives to important policy discussion. Providers are championing this effort across the country; a 2017 review identified 22 health care entities implementing food insecurity screening.[52,53]

Assistance is available through federal and local programs, such as the Supplemental Nutrition Assistance Program (formerly known as "Food Stamps"), Congregate Meals Program, Home-Delivered Meals, Commodity and Supplemental Food Program, Senior Farmers Market Nutrition Program, Child and Adult Care Food Program, and medically tailored meals. In addition, nutrition screening and education may be available at senior centers, schools, and churches (see **Fig. 2**).

Table 3
Nutritional resources

Federal	Other
• https://www.nutrition.gov/subiect/food-assistance-programs/nutrition-programs-seniors	• https://nutritionandaging.org/
• www.cdc.gov	• www.noharm.org
• www.nia.nih.gov/	• www.localharvest.org
• www.choosemyplate.gov	• www.healthvfoodinhealthcare.org
• www.foodsafety.gov	• www.eatright.org
• www.befoodsafe.gov	• www.heart.org
• www.isitdoneyet.gov	• www.aota.org
• www.fruitsandveggiesmatter.gov	• www.foodinsight.org
• www.usda.gov	• www.localharvest.org/csa
• www.cnpp.usda.gov	• www.mavoclinic.com
• www.health.Hov/paHuidelines	• www.mowaa.org
• www.myfoodapedia.gov	• www.nanasp.org
• www.nhlbi.nih.gov	• www.frac.org
• www.niddk.nih.gov	• https://www.hsph.harvard.edu/nutritionsource/
• https://ndb.nal.usda.gov	• https://www.fruitsandveggiesmorematters.org
• https://www.nutrition.va.gov	• https://www.ewg.org/

Table 4
Dietary patterns that support healthy aging

	Description	Features	Health Benefits	Considerations for Older Adults
Mediterranean Diet	Patterned after the dietary traditions and customs of the peoples of the Mediterranean Basin.	High intakes of "healthy" components such as legumes, cereals, fruits, vegetables, and fish as well as a high ratio of monounsaturated to saturated fat and a lower intake of meat and meat products, high-fat milk, and dairy products.[59]	Protective against frailty, functional disability.[57] Associated with slower cognitive decline, lower risk of frailty, and favorable lean body mass in older women.[56,58,59]	[59]None
DASH Diet	Designed to prevent and treat hypertension.	Emphasizes plant-based foods and limits saturated and total fat, cholesterol, and sodium.	Improved markers of cardiovascular health including blood pressure and total cholesterol. Greater cognition in older adults.[60]	None
MIND Diet	Developed to prevent dementia.	A combination of the Mediterranean and DASH diets and specifies natural, plant-based foods and limits animal-source foods and those that are high in saturated fat.	Higher adherence is associated with decreased risk of developing Alzheimer disease and cognitive decline.[61]	None

Table 5
Novel dietary patterns

	Description	Features	Health Benefits	Considerations for Older Adults
Longevity Diet	Developed to assist with weight loss, disease prevention, and extend the lifespan.	A largely plant-based, low protein diet that limits saturated fat and sugar, recommends generous amounts of olive oil and nuts and a multivitamin every 3 d. Advises 2 to 3 meals per day depending on weight and age and confining all eating to within a 24-h period.	Purported clinically demonstrated, beneficial effects on aging and disease risk factors.	Diet may be too low in protein for older adults. The efficacy of fasting diets requires additional investigation. Clinical trials specific to the diet and older adults should be conducted.
Intermittent Fasting	Designed to activate similar biological pathways as calorie restriction to extend the lifespan and improve function in older adults.[67]	Individuals fast (calorie-free beverages ad libitum) and eat (typically unrestricted) for designated (varying) periods.	Weight-loss, changes in weight circumference, increased insulin sensitivity, improved cognitive and physical functioning, and health-related quality of life.[62–66]	Changes in body composition not delineated, that is, unclear if weight loss was due to muscle loss, fat loss, or a combination of both. The efficacy of fasting diets requires additional investigation.
Ketogenic Diet	Established in the 1920s as a therapy for epilepsy.[68,69] Potential therapy for neurodegenerative disorders, insulin resistance, and overweight/obesity.[70,71,77,78]	A very high-fat and low-carbohydrate diet, reducing carbohydrate to ≤10% of consumed energy. The restriction causes a shift from glucose metabolism toward the metabolism of fatty acids yielding ketone bodies as substrates for energy.[72,73]	Associated with improved cognitive performance in elderly adults with Alzheimer disease.[74] Prevention of cognitive decline for those at risk for dementia.[75,76]	Individuals following the ketogenic diet may suffer hypoglycemia and dehydration, muscle loss, and nutrient deficiencies.[74] Further research required.

DIETARY RECOMMENDATIONS THAT SUPPORT HEALTHY AGING

Dietary patterns can be used to inform dietary interventions for older adults. Assessments of dietary patterns have found that diets consistent with current guidelines (including relatively high amounts of vegetables, fruits, whole grains, poultry, fish, and low-fat dairy products) may be associated with superior health status, quality of life, and survival in older adults.[40,41] Dietary recommendations based on foods and cohesive dietary patterns are easier to understand and adopt than numeric amounts of nutrients outlined earlier.[54] Furthermore, dietary patterns may be culturally relevant. Eating is a social activity and should be a pleasurable experience; restrictive diets should be avoided in older adults.[55]

Several plant-based dietary patterns show efficacy preventing frailty and disability and slowing cognitive decline. These plans include the Mediterranean diet, the Dietary Approaches to Stop Hypertension (DASH), and the Mediterranean-DASH Intervention for Neurodegenerative Delay diet, which are summarized in **Table 4**.[56–61]

Table 5 summarizes novel dietary patterns that are being investigated for their efficacy in promoting healthy aging. The longevity diet, intermittent fasting, and the ketogenic diet are receiving attention for the roles they may play in promoting healthy aging.[62–77] Caution should be exercised, as further research, particularly with older adults, is needed.

DISCLOSURE

Dr. Marissa Black was supported by VA Office of Academic Affiliations GRECC Advanced Fellowship in Geriatrics.

REFERENCES

1. Lorenzo-Lopez L, Maseda A, de Labra C, et al. Nutritional determinants of frailty in older adults: a systematic review. BMC Geriatr 2017;17(1):108.
2. GBD 2017 Diet Collaborators. Health effects of dietary risks in 195 countries, 1990-2017: a systematic analysis for the Global Burden of Disease Study 2017. Lancet 2019;393(10184):1958–72.
3. Scarmeas N, Anastasiou CA, Yannakoulia M. Nutrition and prevention of cognitive impairment. Lancet Neurol 2018;17(11):1006–15.
4. Yannakoulia M, Ntanasi E, Anastasiou CA, et al. Frailty and nutrition: from epidemiological and clinical evidence to potential mechanisms. Metabolism 2017;68: 64–76.
5. Wang DD, Li Y, Afshin A, et al. Global improvement in dietary quality could lead to substantial reduction in premature death. J Nutr 2019;149(6):1065–74.
6. Guasch-Ferre M, Satija A, Blondin SA, et al. Meta-analysis of randomized controlled trials of red meat consumption in comparison with various comparison diets on cardiovascular risk factors. Circulation 2019;139(15):1828–45.
7. Buys DR, Roth DL, Ritchie CS, et al. Nutritional risk and body mass index predict hospitalization, nursing home admissions, and mortality in community-dwelling older adults: results from the UAB Study of Aging with 8.5 years of follow-up. J Gerontol A Biol Sci Med Sci 2014;69(9):1146–53.
8. Ramage-Morin PL, Gilmour H, Rotermann M. Nutritional risk, hospitalization and mortality among community-dwelling Canadians aged 65 or older. Health Rep 2017;28(9):17–27.
9. Whitelock E, Ensaff H. On your own: older adults' food choice and dietary habits. Nutrients 2018;10(4):413.

10. Boettger SF, Angersbach B, Klimek CN, et al. Prevalence and predictors of vitamin D-deficiency in frail older hospitalized patients. BMC Geriatr 2018; 18(1):219.
11. Krok-Schoen JL, Archdeacon Price A, Luo M, et al. Low dietary protein intakes and associated dietary patterns and functional limitations in an aging population: a NHANES analysis. J Nutr Health Aging 2019;23(4):338–47.
12. Chapman IM. The anorexia of aging. Clin Geriatr Med 2007;23(4):735–56.
13. Bernstein M, Munoz N. Position of the Academy of Nutrition and Dietetics: food and nutrition for older adults: promoting health and wellness. J Acad Nutr Diet 2012;112(8):1255–77.
14. Evans WJ. Protein nutrition, exercise and aging. J Am Coll Nutr 2004;23(6 Suppl): 601S–9S.
15. Forum NQ. NQF #0421 preventive care and screening: body mass index (BMI) screening and follow-up. 2012. Available at: https://www.qualityforum.org/WorkArea/linkit.aspx?LinkIdentifier=id&ItemID=71112. Accessed May 8, 2020.
16. Kremer S, Bult JH, Mojet J, et al. Food perception with age and its relationship to pleasantness. Chem Senses 2007;32(6):591–602.
17. Boyce JM, Shone GR. Effects of ageing on smell and taste. Postgrad Med J 2006; 82(966):239–41.
18. Murphy C, Schubert CR, Cruickshanks KJ, et al. Prevalence of olfactory impairment in older adults. JAMA 2002;288(18):2307–12.
19. Schiffman SS. Taste and smell losses in normal aging and disease. JAMA 1997; 278(16):1357–62.
20. Tonetti MS, Bottenberg P, Conrads G, et al. Dental caries and periodontal diseases in the ageing population: call to action to protect and enhance oral health and well-being as an essential component of healthy ageing - consensus report of group 4 of the joint EFP/ORCA workshop on the boundaries between caries and periodontal diseases. J Clin Periodontol 2017;44(Suppl 18):S135–44.
21. Dye B, Thornton-Evans G, Li X, et al. Dental caries and tooth loss in adults in the United States, 2011-2012. NCHS Data Brief 2015;(197):197.
22. Eke PI, Dye BA, Wei L, et al. Update on prevalence of periodontitis in adults in the United States: NHANES 2009 to 2012. J Periodontol 2015;86(5):611–22.
23. Gopinath B, Russell J, Sue CM, et al. Olfactory impairment in older adults is associated with poorer diet quality over 5 years. Eur J Nutr 2016;55(3):1081–7.
24. Remond D, Shahar DR, Gille D, et al. Understanding the gastrointestinal tract of the elderly to develop dietary solutions that prevent malnutrition. Oncotarget 2015;6(16):13858–98.
25. Patel KA, Schlundt DG. Impact of moods and social context on eating behavior. Appetite 2001;36(2):111–8.
26. Drewnowski A, Shultz JM. Impact of aging on eating behaviors, food choices, nutrition, and health status. J Nutr Health Aging 2001;5(2):75–9.
27. Ramic E, Pranjic N, Batic-Mujanovic O, et al. The effect of loneliness on malnutrition in elderly population. Med Arh 2011;65(2):92–5.
28. Darmon N, Drewnowski A. Does social class predict diet quality? Am J Clin Nutr 2008;87(5):1107–17.
29. Healthy aging facts. Available at: https://www.ncoa.org/news/resources-for-reporters/get-the-facts/healthy-aging-facts/. Accessed May 31 2019.
30. Roberts AW, Ogunwole SU, Blakeslee L, et al. Census Bureau: the population 65 years and older in the United States: 2016 American community survey reports. 2018. Available at: https://www.census.gov/content/dam/Census/library/publications/2018/acs/ACS-38.pdf. Accessed May 23, 2019.

31. Masnoon N, Shakib S, Kalisch-Ellett L, et al. What is polypharmacy? A systematic review of definitions. BMC Geriatr 2017;17(1):230.

32. Maher RL, Hanlon J, Hajjar ER. Clinical consequences of polypharmacy in elderly. Expert Opin Drug Saf 2014;13(1):57–65.

33. United States Department of Agriculture: Food and Nutrition Service. HEI-2010 total and component scores for children, adults, and older adults during 2011-2012. 2016. Available at: https://fns-prod.azureedge.net/sites/default/files/HEI-2010-During-2011-2012-Oct21-2016.pdf. Accessed November 15, 2019.

34. Roberts SB, Dallal GE. Energy requirements and aging. Public Health Nutr 2005; 8(7A):1028–36.

35. Manini TM. Energy expenditure and aging. Ageing Res Rev 2010;9(1):1–11.

36. Evans WJ. Protein nutrition and resistance exercise. Can J Appl Physiol 2001; 26(Suppl):S141–52.

37. Evans WJ. Exercise and nutritional needs of elderly people: effects on muscle and bone. Gerodontology 1998;15(1):15–24.

38. Dietary reference intakes (DRIs): recommended dietary allowances and adequate intakes, vitamins. US Department of Agriculture. Available at: http://nationalacademies.org/hmd/~/media/Files/Activity%20Files/Nutrition/DRI-Tables/8_Macronutrient%20Summary.pdf. Accessed September 15, 2019.

39. Wright JD, Wang C-Y. Trends in intake of energy and macronutrients in adults from 1999-2000 through 2007-2008. Hyattsville (MD): National Center for Health Statistics; 2010. NCHS data brief, no 49.

40. Ludwig D, Willett W, Volek J, et al. Dietary fat: from foe to friend? Science 2018; 362:764–70.

41. Govindaraju T, Sahle BW, McCaffrey TA, et al. Dietary patterns and quality of life in older adults: a systematic review. Nutrients 2018;10(8).

42. Gonzalez-Campoy JM, St Jeor ST, Castorino K, et al. Clinical practice guidelines for healthy eating for the prevention and treatment of metabolic and endocrine diseases in adults: cosponsored by the American Association of Clinical Endocrinologists/the American College of Endocrinology and the Obesity Society. Endocr Pract 2013;19(Suppl 3):1–82.

43. Hall KD, Ayuketah A, Brychta R, et al. Ultra-processed diets cause excess calorie intake and weight gain: an inpatient randomized controlled trial of Ad Libitum food intake. Cell Metab 2019;30(1):226.

44. Reynolds A, Mann J, Cummings J, et al. Carbohydrate quality and human health: a series of systematic reviews and meta-analyses. Lancet 2019;393(10170): 434–45.

45. Newberry SJ, Chung M, Anderson CAM, et al. Sodium and Potassium Intake: Effects on Chronic Disease Outcomes and Risks. Rockville (MD): RAND Southern California Evidence-based Practice Center: Agency for Healthcare Research and Quality; 2018.

46. Brown IJ, Tzoulaki I, Candeias V, et al. Salt intakes around the world: implications for public health. Int J Epidemiol 2009;38(3):791–813.

47. National Council on Aging. Malnutrition screen and assessment tools. Available at: https://www.ncoa.org/assesssments-tools/malnutrition-screening-assessment-tools/. Accessed April 15, 2019.

48. Miller MP. Best questions and tools for quickly assessing your patient's dietary health: towards evidence-based determination of nutritional counseling need in the general medical interview. Available at: https://escholarship.org/uc/item/9s03p43r#main. Accessed April 15, 2019.

49. Seligman H. Hunger is a Health Issue: Equipping the Anti-Hunger Community for Success. Paper presented at: National Anti-Hunger Policy Conference 2019; Washington, DC, February 29th -March 3rd, 2019.

50. Pooler JA, Hartline-Grafton H, DeBor M, et al. Food insecurity: a key social determinant of health for older adults. J Am Geriatr Soc 2019;67(3):421–4.

51. Pooler JA, Hoffman VA, Karva FJ. Primary care providers' perspectives on screening older adult patients for food insecurity. J Aging Soc Policy 2018; 30(1):1–23.

52. Gundersen C, Engelhard EE, Crumbaugh AS, et al. Brief assessment of food insecurity accurately identifies high-risk US adults. Public Health Nutr 2017; 20(8):1367–71.

53. Lundeen EA, Siegel KR, Calhoun H, et al. Clinical-community partnerships to identify patients with food insecurity and address food needs. Prev Chronic Dis 2017;14:E113.

54. Cespedes EM, Hu FB. Dietary patterns: from nutritional epidemiologic analysis to national guidelines. Am J Clin Nutr 2015;101(5):899–900.

55. Locher JL, Robinson CO, Roth DL, et al. The effect of the presence of others on caloric intake in homebound older adults. J Gerontol A Biol Sci Med Sci 2005; 60(11):1475–8.

56. Ward RE, Orkaby AR, Chen J, et al. Association between diet quality and frailty prevalence in the physicians' health study. J Am Geriatr Soc 2019;68(4):770–6.

57. Silva R, Pizato N, da Mata F, et al. Mediterranean diet and musculoskeletal-functional outcomes in community-dwelling older people: a systematic review and meta-analysis. J Nutr Health Aging 2018;22(6):655–63.

58. Feart C, Samieri C, Barberger-Gateau P. Mediterranean diet and cognitive function in older adults. Curr Opin Clin Nutr Metab Care 2010;13(1):14–8.

59. Nikolov J, Spira D, Aleksandrova K, et al. Adherence to a mediterranean-style diet and appendicular lean mass in community-dwelling older people: results from the Berlin aging study II. J Gerontol A Biol Sci Med Sci 2016;71(10): 1315–21.

60. Wengreen H, Munger RG, Cutler A, et al. Prospective study of dietary approaches to stop hypertension- and mediterranean-style dietary patterns and age-related cognitive change: the cache county study on memory, health and aging. Am J Clin Nutr 2013;98(5):1263–71.

61. McEvoy CT, Guyer H, Langa KM, et al. Neuroprotective diets are associated with better cognitive function: the health and retirement study. J Am Geriatr Soc 2017; 65(8):1857–62.

62. Heilbronn LK, Smith SR, Martin CK, et al. Alternate-day fasting in nonobese subjects: effects on body weight, body composition, and energy metabolism. Am J Clin Nutr 2005;81(1):69–73.

63. Harvie MN, Pegington M, Mattson MP, et al. The effects of intermittent or continuous energy restriction on weight loss and metabolic disease risk markers: a randomized trial in young overweight women. Int J Obes (Lond) 2011;35(5):714–27.

64. Harvie M, Wright C, Pegington M, et al. The effect of intermittent energy and carbohydrate restriction v. daily energy restriction on weight loss and metabolic disease risk markers in overweight women. Br J Nutr 2013;110(8):1534–47.

65. Horie NC, Serrao VT, Simon SS, et al. Cognitive effects of intentional weight loss in elderly obese individuals with mild cognitive impairment. J Clin Endocrinol Metab 2016;101(3):1104–12.

66. Leclerc E, Trevizol AP, Grigolon RB, et al. The effect of caloric restriction on working memory in healthy non-obese adults. CNS Spectr 2020;25(1):2–8.

67. Anton SD, Lee SA, Donahoo WT, et al. The effects of time restricted feeding on overweight, older adults: a pilot study. Nutrients 2019;11(7):1500.
68. Pinto A, Bonucci A, Maggi E, et al. Anti-oxidant and anti-inflammatory activity of ketogenic diet: new perspectives for neuroprotection in Alzheimer's disease. Antioxidants (Basel) 2018;7(5):63.
69. Huttenlocher PR. Ketonemia and seizures: metabolic and anticonvulsant effects of two ketogenic diets in childhood epilepsy. Pediatr Res 1976;10(5):536–40.
70. Zhao Z, Lange DJ, Voustianiouk A, et al. A ketogenic diet as a potential novel therapeutic intervention in amyotrophic lateral sclerosis. BMC Neurosci 2006; 7:29.
71. Augustin K, Khabbush A, Williams S, et al. Mechanisms of action for the medium-chain triglyceride ketogenic diet in neurological and metabolic disorders. Lancet Neurol 2018;17(1):84–93.
72. Taylor MK, Sullivan DK, Mahnken JD, et al. Feasibility and efficacy data from a ketogenic diet intervention in Alzheimer's disease. Alzheimers Dement (NY) 2018;4:28–36.
73. Taylor MK, Swerdlow RH, Burns JM, et al. An experimental ketogenic diet for Alzheimer disease was nutritionally dense and rich in vegetables and Avocado. Curr Dev Nutr 2019;3(4):nzz003.
74. Rusek M, Pluta R, Ulamek-Koziol M, et al. Ketogenic diet in Alzheimer's disease. Int J Mol Sci 2019;20(16):3892.
75. Nagpal R, Neth BJ, Wang S, et al. Modified Mediterranean-ketogenic diet modulates gut microbiome and short-chain fatty acids in association with Alzheimer's disease markers in subjects with mild cognitive impairment. EBioMedicine 2019; 47:529–42.
76. Neth BJ, Mintz A, Whitlow C, et al. Modified ketogenic diet is associated with improved cerebrospinal fluid biomarker profile, cerebral perfusion, and cerebral ketone body uptake in older adults at risk for Alzheimer's disease: a pilot study. Neurobiol Aging 2020;86:54–63.
77. Vanitallie TB, Nonas C, Di Rocco A, et al. Treatment of Parkinson disease with diet-induced hyperketonemia: a feasibility study. Neurology 2005;64(4):728–30.
78. Reger MA, Henderson ST, Hale C, et al. Effects of beta-hydroxybutyrate on cognition in memory-impaired adults. Neurobiol Aging 2004;25(3):311–4.

Physical Activity and Healthy Aging

Elizabeth Eckstrom, MD, MPH*, Suvi Neukam, DO, Leah Kalin, MD, Jessica Wright, PA-C

KEYWORDS

- Healthy aging • Older adults • Exercise • Physical activity

KEY POINTS

- Physical activity prevents sarcopenia, osteoporosis, falls, and many other conditions that hinder healthy aging.
- Physical activity improves mobility, cognition, and independent functioning.
- Older adults benefit from aerobic, strength, flexibility, and balance training.

INTRODUCTION

Aging is the progressive deterioration at the cellular, tissue, and organ level that leads to loss of homeostasis, decreased ability to adapt to internal or external stimuli, and increased vulnerability to disease and death. Visible imprints of aging are loss of quantity and pigmentation of hair, diminished height, decreased muscle mass, and thin wrinkled skin. But it is not as bad as it sounds. The human body is an amazing machine. Meet Man Kaur, a 101-year-old winner of the World Masters Games in New Zealand, where she completed the 100-m dash in just 74 seconds. She is the oldest woman to achieve this feat. Kaur's accomplishment is even more remarkable in that she only began her running career at the age of 96. In this article, we explore how the aging process affects our bodies and how exercise positively impacts these processes.

CHANGES TO THE MUSCULOSKELETAL SYSTEM WITH AGE

The musculoskeletal system is a diverse group of tissues including muscles, bones, tendons, ligaments, and cartilage, which work together to maintain physical function. Normal physiologic aging influences each of these tissues in different ways. With age, muscle fibers, in particular the type II or fast twitch fibers, shrink in size and number. This results in a decrease in strength and muscle tone. Normal physiologic aging is associated with loss of lean muscle mass, an increase in lipofuscin and other cellular

Division of General Internal Medicine & Geriatrics, Department of Medicine, Oregon Health & Science University, 3181 Southwest Sam Jackson Park Road, L475, Portland, OR 97239, USA
* Corresponding author.
E-mail address: eckstrom@ohsu.edu

Clin Geriatr Med 36 (2020) 671–683
https://doi.org/10.1016/j.cger.2020.06.009
0749-0690/20/© 2020 Elsevier Inc. All rights reserved.

waste products, and fat deposits. This process is known as sarcopenia. Muscle mass actually begins to decline around the age of 35. Aging muscle tissue is more vulnerable to injury and slower to recover from injuries. Over time, cartilage loses hydration and increases in calcium content. When excessive, this can lead to osteoarthritis. There is also increased stiffness of ligaments and tendons, which leads to less mobile joints and slowed, more limited body movements. Bone mineral density also decreases with normal aging, and can result in osteoporosis, leading to increased risk for fractures. Lastly, an increasingly recognized geriatric syndrome, frailty, is a pathologic syndrome of physiologic decline in late life characterized by increased susceptibility to adverse health outcomes. Frail older adults are less able to adapt to stressors, such as infection or trauma caused by narrower physiologic reserves from accumulation of chronic conditions. This leads to increased risk for many adverse health outcomes, such as falls, need for institutionalization, disability, and death. Although frailty is associated with older age, it is not synonymous with old age, nor is frailty a normal aging process. Many older adults remain vigorous throughout their life span.

Osteoarthritis, sarcopenia, osteoporosis, falls, and frailty are not inevitable consequences of aging. In fact, each of these is largely preventable through physical activity. Numerous studies have demonstrated the positive effects of exercise on the aging musculoskeletal system and the negative consequences of inactivity. In one study, inactivity, which was defined as 10 days of continuous bed rest in healthy older subjects, was associated with a 30% reduction in muscle protein synthesis, a 1.5-kg loss of lean mass (mostly from the lower extremities), and a 16% decrement in lower extremity strength.[1] Although exercise does not slow loss of muscle fibers, it can slow loss of muscle mass by increasing the size of remaining fibers. Strength training in particular improves muscle force and metabolic capacity, increases glycogen storage, and enhances oxidative enzyme activity. In the next sections, we explore how exercise positively impacts the musculoskeletal system; improves pain; decreases risk for falls; and improves cognition, sleep, and other important functions. We focus primarily on exercise benefits to promote optimal mobility and independence, which are truly the heart of healthy aging. Like Man Kaur, all older adults have the ability to maintain and improve physical fitness into very old age.

BENEFITS OF EXERCISE FOR HEALTHY AGING

Current estimates suggest that the population of adults 65 and older will increase from 46.2 million to approximately 98 million by the year 2060. If our expanding older adult population is to continue to contribute to society, we need to optimize healthy aging for the entire population. Regular daily activity is critical to healthy aging and reducing frailty and risk for falls, maintaining function, and reducing premature morbidity.[2,3] Exercise promotes a longer life span, the amount of time we live, and a longer health span, the amount of healthy time we live.[4] Exercise is key to the prevention and management of many conditions common in the adult population including hypertension, diabetes, obesity, insomnia, depression, and anxiety.

Improved Mobility

Mobility is the ability to ambulate without assistance and is critical to independence for older adults. Major mobility disability, as defined by the ability to walk less than 400 m in 15 minutes without sitting, the help of another person, or use of a walker, is reduced by regular participation in moderate-level physical activity, including aerobic, resistance, and flexibility training exercises.[5]

Reduced Risk of Sarcopenia and Frailty

Sarcopenia is highly correlated with frailty. The key to preventing and reversing sarcopenia is building muscle. Strength training, aerobic exercise, and flexibility exercise can increase muscle strength and size, resulting in increased functional capacity and gait speed.[6]

Osteoporosis Prevention and Management

Osteoporosis affects up to 200 million people worldwide, and is associated with significant morbidity and mortality, especially in older adults who fall.[7] High-impact exercise, resistance training, and muscle strengthening all promote bone turnover and, in doing so, improve bone strength and prevent and manage osteoporosis.[8,9] Physical activity is also effective at reducing fractures.[10] A 2011 Cochrane Review summarized the evidence in the following way, "of 100 postmenopausal women who exercise, seven will have a fracture, compared to 11 in 100 who don't exercise."[11]

Fall Prevention

Approximately one-third of people older than the age of 65 fall annually. Fall risks include reduced muscle strength, impaired reflexes, decreased proprioception, and loss of mobility, all of which are common with aging. Balance training, flexibility training, strength and resistance training, and tai chi improve agility, coordination, and balance and help prevent or reverse these changes. Each of these interventions has demonstrated a reduction in falls.[12] Overall, exercise reduces the number of falls over time by 23%, and reduces the total number of older adults who experience one or more falls.[11]

Pain

Pain is reported by up to 62% of adults older than the age 75 with conditions including rheumatoid arthritis, osteoarthritis, fibromyalgia, low back pain, claudication, spinal stenosis, neuropathy, and visceral pain.[13] Normal aging may increase pain facilitation and reduce capacity to inhibit pain inputs. Frequent movement is key to the prevention and treatment of pain. Aerobic, strength, flexibility, core or balance training programs, yoga, Pilates, and tai chi have been shown to reduce quantitative pain recordings and reported pain severity scores.[13,14] Physical function is higher in participants of these activities, presumably because of reduced pain. Older adults who engage in moderate to vigorous physical activity actually experience "exercise-induced hypoalgesia" and an increased pain threshold. Exercise training and regular daily activity may prevent chronic pain via reduced pain sites and pain intensity.[15] Daily physical activity reduces lower extremity osteoarthritic pain and stiffness along with improving overall functional capacity.[16]

Cognition and Memory

Prospective studies identify physical inactivity as one of the greatest risk factors for developing Alzheimer disease (AD). Increased physical activity can reverse this risk. Let us explore how.

Exercise increases blood flow to the brain, which promotes neurogenesis.[17] In older adults at risk for AD, participation in exercise helps maintain volume of the hippocampus, the part of the brain responsible for processing various forms of memory. Moderate physical activity also increases glucose metabolism in areas of the brain that are hypometabolic in AD.[18] Reduction in gross cerebral changes typical of dementia (macroinfarcts, nigral neuronal loss, and white matter pathology) correlate with increased levels of total daily activity.[19]

Muscle strengthening and aerobic activity improves performance on cognitive tests and reduces risk of AD. One prospective cohort study found that increased extremity and axial strength resulted in a 43% lower risk of developing AD and a slower rate of observed cognitive decline.[20] Individuals resistant to hitting the gym need not be discouraged; cognitive improvement has been observed with routine daily movement.[21] Exercise may also reduce the often devastating and debilitating neuropsychiatric symptoms that accompany AD.[17] It seems that physical activity is not only good for the body but also the mind.

TYPES OF EXERCISE

Multiple national guidelines recommend a multimodal exercise prescription as the single most beneficial intervention to improve health in older adults (**Table 1**). This should include aerobic exercise, resistance training, and balance and flexibility exercises.[3]

Aerobic Exercise

Aerobic exercise reduces risk of cardiovascular disease, improves glucose tolerance and bone mineral density, decreases inflammation and oxidative stress, and improves mitochondrial biogenesis and protein synthesis in skeletal muscle.[22] The type of aerobic exercise is not as important as the frequency, duration, and effort. Even doing regular leisure activities has positive cardiovascular benefits in frail older adults, but aerobic activities that include moderate- and vigorous-intensity exercise have a more significant reduction in mortality.[23] The US Department of Health recommends older adults engage in at least 150 minutes per week of moderate-intensity exercise or 75 minutes per week of vigorous-intensity exercise. Moderate-intensity exercise is defined as aerobic exercise that is performed at a perceived effort at a 5 or 6 level, where 0 is defined as the effort of sitting and 10 is defined as maximal effort. Vigorous intensity is a perceived effort of 7 or 8 on the same scale.[3]

Walking is the most popular physical activity enjoyed by older adults likely because it is low-cost and accessible, and is done alone or in groups, outside and indoors.[24] The widespread availability and popularity of pedometers, or step counters, have likely also contributed to the popularity of walking. Walking is most valuable when performed at a moderate to vigorous intensity.

Table 1
Benefits of different types of exercise to various older adult–specific conditions

	Aerobic Exercise	Strength Exercise	Balance and Flexibility Exercise	Highest Impact Recommendation
Mobility	✔	✔	✔	Well-balanced
Sarcopenia	✔	✔	✔	exercise program!
Osteoporosis	✔[a]	✔	✔	
Falls	✔	✔	✔	
Pain	✔	✔	✔	
Cognition	✔	✔	✔	

[a] Only if weight-bearing or impact aerobic exercise.

Water-based aerobic activity has been widely supported as an aerobic exercise that is easier for people with osteoarthritis to participate in. Individuals who participated in a walking program performed in water were able to increase their walking intensity compared with a control group on land presumably because of less joint pain, and the heat dissipation offered by the aquatic environment. These physiologic phenomenon may make water-based aerobic exercise beneficial for individuals who have a decreased exercise tolerance and are unable to achieve moderate- or vigorous-intensity exercise because of increased heart rate demands and/or joint pain.[25] Water reduces the impact of gravity, so water-based exercise does not help prevent or treat osteoporosis.

Cycling can help older adults with arthritis, Parkinson disease, and other conditions achieve moderate to vigorous exercise. Already fairly fit older women were able to improve their muscle strength using a cycling program and led to increases in walking speeds and improvements in functional abilities.[26] Cycling allows individuals to slowly increase their effort and duration over time, which may be particularly useful in chronic conditions that make aerobic exercise challenging, such as emphysema or congestive heart failure. There was no difference in strength and functional outcomes in patients who cycled at a higher speed but lower resistance compared with the group who cycled at a higher resistance and lower speeds.

Although achieving a moderate or vigorous level of activity may be easier with some activities compared with others, finding activities that one enjoys is equally important. Aerobic activity may not only be a way for older adults to reduce frailty and improve activities of daily living, it may also be a means to avert social isolation and boredom. Group exercise has psychosocial benefits that may help to improve adherence and enjoyment of aerobic activities for older adults.

Resistance Exercise

Strength training involves using resistance to generate muscular contraction, thereby increasing the ability to produce muscular force. Strength training not only leads to increased muscle hypertrophy, but also increased anaerobic endurance, increased bone density,[27] lowered insulin resistance, improved mobility, decreased incidence of frailty, and reduction in all-cause mortality.[28] Examples include free weight training (barbells, kettlebells, and dumbbells), bodyweight training (using the trainee's own bodyweight to produce resistance), resistance bands, and weight training machines. The best programs focus on multijoint exercises, such as dead-lifts, squats, and presses that involve all the major muscle groups, working them through a full range of motion. Studies show that when combined with proper nutrition, strength training is perhaps the single most effective intervention to prevent sarcopenia.[29]

Most of the decline in skeletal muscle mass associated with aging is related to the disproportionate denervation and subsequent loss of the type II, or fast-twitch muscle fibers. The resultant decrease in muscular force associated with aging is called dynapenia.[30] Fortunately, long-term resistance training has been shown to stimulate existing type II muscle fibers. Strength training should be systematically planned in a rationally progressive manner over an extended time. Strength training cannot be accomplished by intermittent bouts of exercise. This is called progressive overload: application of a training load, allowance for recovery, and incremental increase in the training load, which leads to adaption and increased performance over time.[31] When carried out properly using a carefully planned program, well-titrated loads, and rational progression, strength training is safe. However, when programming or technique are poor, this can lead to injury.

Table 2
Well-balanced, evidence-based exercise programs for community-dwelling older adults

Name of Program	Program Description
Tai Chi for Arthritis	Evidence-based falls prevention program that uses tai chi to improve balance, flexibility, strength, and mobility. Classes are 1 h and intended to be twice weekly for 8 wk. Participants must attend an in-person class once per week but can do the exercises on their own with an instructional video. Classes seem to be available throughout the United States. Cost may be variable. https://www.ncoa.org/resources/tai-chi-arthritis-program-information-guidance/
Tai chi: moving for better balance	Evidence-based exercise program designed to improve strength, balance, flexibility, and mobility through tai chi exercises. Classes are 12 wk, participants meet twice weekly for 60–90 min plus are expected to do home exercises for 2 or more hours per week. Program is based in senior centers, gyms, and YMCAs across the country. Research has shown improvements in balance, strength, flexibility, mobility, and a decrease in fall risk in participants. https://www.ncoa.org/resources/ymca-moving-better-balance-program-summary/
EnhanceFitness (formerly Lifetime Fitness Program)	Focuses on low-impact CV fitness, balance work, strength training, and stretching. Program has been shown to reduce risk of falls resulting in medical care and improve TUG, chair stand, and arm curl measurements in a couple of studies. Low cost. Classes meet 3 times/wk, sessions are 1-h long. Available in 40 states. https://www.ncoa.org/resources/enhancefitness-program-summary/
First Step to Active Health	Self-guided program that is designed to improve physical fitness for people with chronic disease. Four-step routine to improve aerobic capacity, flexibility, balance, and strength. Materials are available online or in print. Exercises can be done individually but may also be done in a group setting. Two pilot studies used the Senior Fitness Test to assess before and after results. Both studies showed an improvement in physical fitness. http://firststeptoactivehealth.com/youcan/index.htm
Fit and Strong!	Program that combines aerobic walking, strength training, flexibility training, and health education. Also uses group problem solving/education and some individualized instruction. Targeted at adults with lower extremity OA, program is designed to improve lower extremity stiffness and joint pain. Program is 90 min, 3 times per week for 8 wk. RCT showed that participants that completed the program had increased exercise tolerance, increased physical activity, reduced joint pain and stiffness. A larger study was done with the same program and got similar results and improvements in timed-stands test, mobility, and improved depression and anxiety over the study period (18 mo). https://www.ncoa.org/resources/program-summary-fit-and-strong/

(continued on next page)

Table 2 (continued)	
Name of Program	**Program Description**
Go4Life	Program sponsored by the NIA addressing endurance (ie, aerobic), strength training, balance, and flexibility exercises. Education materials are free to patients either on the NIA Web site or in print. Materials describe specific exercises in each category and recommended frequency and duration. Includes tools for setting goals and tracking progress. https://go4life.nia.nih.gov/

Abbreviations: CV, cardiovascular; NIA, National Institute on Aging; OA, osteoarthritis; RCT, randomized controlled trial; TUG, Timed Up and Go.

Strength training programs must be highly individualized for older adults. Exercises should be tailored to what the older individual can perform safely, making adjustments for mobility restrictions and being especially mindful of recovery periods. Compared with their younger cohorts, older adults may require more frequent exposure to resistance loading to build and maintain strength, may progress more slowly, require smaller increases in loading, and plateau earlier than younger subjects. The overall training frequency required for progress loading is highly individualized. Beginners should train 2 to 3 days per week, and loading exercises should range within 8 to 12 repetitions at maximum weight. The number of sets should be increased slowly over multiple training sessions (2%–10% once the individual can perform the current workload for 1–2 repetitions more than the goal number of repetitions).[32] We recommend referring older adult trainees to a strength and conditioning professional with experience working with older adults, but if that is not possible, the mantra "start low, go slow—but go" fits.

Balance and Flexibility Exercise

Tai chi is probably the best studied of the balance and flexibility exercises, and has numerous benefits for healthy aging. In multiple randomized controlled trials, tai chi performed for 1 hour twice per week reduces falls by at least 50%.[33,34] Tai chi emphasizes control over one's body mass displacement, postural alignment, and range of motion of lower extremity joints and muscles, increasing lower extremity strength, postural stability, and improving balance.[34] It reduces pain in knee osteoarthritis[35] and fibromyalgia,[36] probably through improved core strength and flexibility. It improves executive function (important for remaining independent in the community),[37] possibly through the requirement of dual tasking (movement plus needing to remember the moves). It increases walk time in people with congestive heart failure,[38] improves sleep quality,[39] and has many other healthy aging benefits. Tai chi is truly an activity in which all older adults should participate. Yoga has much less evidence to support its efficacy for healthy aging in older adults, but early studies show it may be effective to improve sleep quality, depression, and overall health status in older adults.[40]

Counseling Older Adults for Regular Daily Activity

There is no age or stage of frailty that precludes regular daily activity. Indeed, "healthy aging" no longer implies being lucky enough to live to an old age without accumulating major medical illnesses but rather optimizing quality of life, mobility, independence,

Table 3
Evidence-based exercise programs that are home-based or designed for more frail older adults

Name of Program	Program Description
Active Choices	6-mo telephone-based exercise program. Program is individualized and is designed to promote long-term participation in exercise with minimal face-to-face contact. Initial visit is a face-to-face session with a health educator. Exercise program is made based on patient's level of functioning and personal preference. Patient is given tools to track progress. Follow-up calls are initially made weekly then transition to biweekly then monthly. Program is 6 mo. Study performed with cardiac rehabilitation patients showed similar outcomes of increased functional capacity and exercise adherence and similar low rates for reinfarction in patients who participated in the Active Choice program compared with a group-based, structured exercise class. https://www.ncoa.org/resources/program-summary-active-choices/
Geri-fit	Progressive resistance strength training exercise program. Exercises are performed in chairs with optional standing. Classes are twice weekly for 45 min. Multiple studies have been performed that show improvements mainly in postural stability, which is believed to be directly related to balance. https://www.gerifit.com/
Healthy Moving for Aging Well (Health Moves)	Home-based exercise program targeted toward frail, high-risk patients in community-based care management programs. Uses simple seated and standing exercises and provides counseling/support to foster lifestyle changes using the Stages of Change model. Participants are encouraged to do their exercises 3–5 d per week, multiple times per day. Motivational telephone coaches contact clients weekly or biweekly for a 3-mo period. Studies have shown continued participation in physical exercise after 6 mo and a reduction in number of falls and improvement in upper and lower extremity strength. https://www.ncoa.org/resources/program-summary-healthy-moves-for-aging-well/

(continued on next page)

Table 3 (continued)	
Name of Program	Program Description
Walk with Ease	Program targeted toward people with arthritis. It is a 6-wk walking program with either a self-guided format or a community format. Program is through the Arthritis Foundation and includes an individualized walking plan, stretching exercises, and heart-rate monitoring techniques. Materials were developed from previous research that was shown to improve physical activity, increase walking distance and speed, and to decrease pain. https://www.arthritis.org/living-with-arthritis/tools-resources/walk-with-ease/
Bingocize	A bingo-based game that combines exercise and health education. Can be done in a group setting but also available on a mobile app. Game includes some exercises for upper and lower extremities but also includes questions regarding health and fall prevention. Research demonstrated increases in upper and lower body strength compared with control group and improvements in walking gait speed and overall health knowledge. https://www.ncoa.org/resources/bingocize-program-summary/

engagement, and purpose despite physical and mental challenges that arise. The first counseling strategy for physical activity is simply this: older adults can, and should, work to improve their fitness no matter what stage of health or frailty they are at. This does not mean establishing a new world record in the 100-m dash at 101 as Man Kaur did. It means taking a measured approach to finding a well-balanced exercise program that works for each older adult.

First, discover what your patient likes to do for exercise, or what they enjoyed in their past (if they are not currently exercising). Listen to the patient and use motivational interviewing techniques to establish their life goals (eg, being able to babysit grandchildren) and their preferred activities (swimming if they used to enjoy swimming) and then craft a graduated activity program to meet their goals.[41] Use the Stages of Change model to assess their current motivation to be active and target your recommendations to the stage they are at (eg, if they are in precontemplation, simply ask them to consider if there are things in their life that they would like to do but may not be able to do because of their mobility limitations; if they are in the preparation stage help them to set realistic goals to try out activity, such as attending a local tai chi class just to see what it is like).[42] Some older adults have always hated exercise, but might do some sit to stand exercises with a grandchild.

Next, tailor your exercise recommendations to the patient's current health status. Most older adults can begin a graduated exercise program without any special evaluation (eg, an exercise treadmill test) if they start slowly and progress gradually, such as 10 minutes of slow walking gradually working up to 30 minutes of brisk walking over a month or two. For patients with uncontrolled hypertension, congestive heart failure,

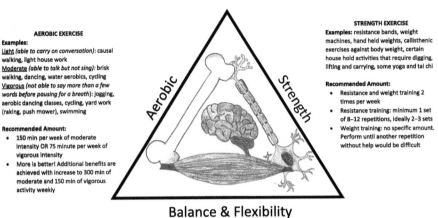

AEROBIC EXERCISE

Examples:
Light *(able to carry on conversation)*: casual walking, light house work
Moderate *(able to talk but not sing)*: brisk walking, dancing, water aerobics, cycling
Vigorous *(not able to say more than a few words before pausing for a breath)*: jogging, aerobic dancing classes, cycling, yard work (raking, push mower), swimming

Recommended Amount:
- 150 min per week of moderate intensity OR 75 minute per week of vigorous intensity
- More is better! Additional benefits are achieved with increase to 300 min of moderate and 150 min of vigorous activity weekly

STRENGTH EXERCISE

Examples: resistance bands, weight machines, hand held weights, callisthenic exercises against body weight, certain house hold activities that require digging, lifting and carrying, some yoga and tai chi

Recommended Amount:
- Resistance and weight training 2 times per week
- Resistance training: minimum 1 set of 8–12 repetitions, ideally 2–3 sets
- Weight training: no specific amount. Perform until another repetition without help would be difficult

Balance & Flexibility

BALANCE & FLEXIBILITY EXERCISE

Examples: tai chi, sit to stands, walking variations (backward, sideways, heel and toe), stretching

Recommended Amount:
- Balance: minimum 2 times per week participation in a standardized program demonstrated to reduce falls (Ex. Tai Chi)
- Flexibility: minimum 2 times per week

Fig. 1. Recommendations for a well-balanced exercise regimen. (*Data from* Mora J, Valencia WM. Exercise and older adults. Clin Geriatr Med. 2018;34(1):145–62; and Lee PG, Jackson EA, Richardson CR. Exercise prescriptions in older adults. Am Fam Physician. 2017;95(7):425–32.)

angina, or chronic obstructive pulmonary disease, it may be prudent to do further cardiopulmonary testing before starting regular exercise. If your patient is very frail and homebound, the Otago home health PT intervention to reduce fall risk may be a great choice.[43] Maybe they can start doing tai chi sitting in a chair (try Suman Barkhas' You Tube seated tai chi video). If they are currently walking 5 days per week but doing nothing else, get their thoughts on adding a yoga or tai chi class. It might take months to work up to a well-balanced exercise program (and might take months to really feel the benefits; here is where your good cheerleading can help maintain motivation), but you can help your patients celebrate small successes along the way and keep them engaged in making progress. It is always a great reminder that the greater one's frailty and deconditioning, the faster they will improve with regular exercise.[44]

SUMMARY

Regular physical activity is one of the most important components of healthy aging. It prevents or helps manage most of the key challenges older adults face: pain, decreased mobility, frailty, cognitive impairment, and many others. No one is too old or too frail to begin a regular activity program. Providers and all members of the health care team and community-based organizations can and should assist older adults in finding an optimal physical activity program for them. We have compiled evidence-based exercise programs that combine well-balanced exercise interventions (**Table 2** for more fit community-dwelling older adults, **Table 3** for more frail older adults). Resources were chosen based on their national availability and with an eye to cost. We also include a summary of the specific recommendations around type, duration, and frequency of activity for each component of a well-balanced exercise program (**Fig. 1**). Together with our older adult patients, we can all enjoy a healthier old age through the power of regular physical activity.

DISCLOSURE

The authors have nothing to disclose.

REFERENCES

1. Kortebein P, Symons B, Ferrando A, et al. Functional impact of 10 days of bed rest in healthy older adults. J Gerontol A Biol Sci Med Sci 2008;63:1076–81.
2. Theou O, Stathokostas L, Roland K, et al. The effectiveness of exercise interventions for the management of frailty: a systematic review. J Aging Res 2011;2011:569194.
3. Mora J, Valencia WM. Exercise and older adults. Clin Geriatr Med 2018;34(1):145–62.
4. Kaeberlein M. How healthy is the healthspan concept? Geroscience 2018;40:361–4.
5. Pahor M, Guralnik JM, Ambrosius WT, et al. Effect of structured physical activity on prevention of major mobility disability in older adults: the LIFE study randomized clinical trial. JAMA 2014;311(23):2387–96.
6. Liguori I, Russo G, Aran L, et al. Sarcopenia: assessment of disease burden and strategies to improve outcomes. Clin Interv Aging 2018;13:913–27.
7. International Osteoporosis Foundation. Available at: https://www.iofbonehealth.org/epidemiology IOF https://www.iofbonehealth.org/epidemiology. Accessed October 1, 2019.
8. Howe TE, Shea B, Dawson LJ, et al. Exercise for preventing and treating osteoporosis in postmenopausal women. Cochrane Database Syst Rev 2011;(7):CD000333.
9. Daly RM, Dalla Via J, Duckham RL, et al. Exercise for the prevention of osteoporosis in postmenopausal women: an evidence-based guide to the optimal prescription. Braz J Phys Ther 2019;23(2):170–80.
10. Kemmler W, Häberle L, von Stengel S. Effects of exercise on fracture reduction in older adults: a systematic review and meta-analysis. Osteoporos Int 2013;24:1937.
11. Sherrington C, Fairhall NJ, Wallbank GK, et al. Exercise for preventing falls in older people living in the community. Cochrane Database Syst Rev 2019;(1):CD012424.
12. Sherrington C, Michaleff ZA, Fairhall N, et al. Exercise to prevent falls in older adults: an updated systematic review and meta-analysis. Br J Sports Med 2017;51:1750–8.
13. Geneen LJ, Moore R, Clarke C, et al. Physical activity and exercise for chronic pain in adults: an overview of Cochrane Reviews. Cochrane Database Syst Rev 2017;(4):CD011279.
14. Naugle KM, Ohlman T, Naugle KE, et al. Physical activity behavior predicts endogenous pain modulation in older adults. Pain 2017;158(3):383–90.
15. Hirase T, Kataoka H, Inokuchi S, et al. Effects of exercise training combined with increased physical activity to prevent chronic pain in community-dwelling older adults: a preliminary randomized controlled trial. Pain Res Manag 2018;2018:2132039.
16. Fransen M, McConnell S, Hernandez-Molina G, et al. Exercise for osteoarthritis of the hip. Cochrane Database Syst Rev 2014;(4):CD007912.
17. Cass SP. Alzheimer's disease and exercise: a literature review. Curr Sports Med Rep 2017;16(1):19–22.

18. Dougherty RJ, Schultz SA, Kirby TK, et al. Moderate physical activity is associated with cerebral glucose metabolism in adults at risk for Alzheimer's disease. J Alzheimers Dis 2017;58(4):1089–97.

19. Buchman AS, Dawe RJ, Yu L, et al. Brain pathology is related to total daily physical activity in older adults. Neurology 2018;90(21):e1911–9.

20. Boyle PA, Buchman AS, Wilson RS, et al. Association of muscle strength with the risk of Alzheimer disease and the rate of cognitive decline in community-dwelling older persons. Arch Neurol 2009;66(11):1339–44.

21. Buchman AS, Boyle PA, Yu L, et al. Total daily physical activity and the risk of AD and cognitive decline in older adults. Neurology 2012;78(17):1323–9.

22. Ikenaga M, Yamada Y, Kose Y, et al. Effects of a 12-week, short-interval, intermittent, low-intensity, slow-jogging program on skeletal muscle, fat infiltration, and fitness in older adults: randomized controlled trial. Eur J Appl Physiol 2017; 117:7–15.

23. Samitz G, Egger M, Zwahlen M. Domains of physical activity and all-cause mortality: systematic review and dose-response meta-analysis of cohort studies. Int J Epidemiol 2011;40(5):1382–400.

24. Reitlo LS, Sandbakk SB, Viken H, et al. Exercise patterns in older adults instructed to follow moderate- or high-intensity exercise protocol-the generation 100 study. BMC Geriatr 2018;18:208.

25. Handa S, Masuki S, Ohshio T, et al. Target intensity and interval walking training in water to enhance physical fitness in middle-aged and older women: a randomised controlled study. Eur J Appl Physiol 2016;116:203–15.

26. Macaluso A, Young A, Gibb K, et al. Cycling as a novel approach to resistance training increases muscle strength, power and selected functional abilities in healthy older women. J Appl Physiol 2003;95:2544–53.

27. Kelley GA, Kelley KS, Tran ZV. Resistance training and bone mineral density in women: a meta-analysis of controlled trials. Am J Phys Med Rehabil 2001; 80(1):65.

28. Kodama S, Saito K, Tanaka S, et al. Cardiorespiratory fitness as a quantitative predictor of all-cause mortality and cardiovascular events in healthy men and women: a meta-analysis. JAMA 2009;301:2024.

29. Waters D, Baumgartner R, Garry P, et al. Advantages of dietary, exercise-related, and therapeutic interventions to prevent and treat sarcopenia in adult patients: an update. Clin Interv Aging 2010;5:259–70.

30. Manini TM, Clark BC. Dynapenia and aging: an update. J Gerontol A Biol Sci Med Sci 2012;67A(1):28–40.

31. Baraki A, Feigenbaum J, Sullivan J. Practical guidelines for implementing a strength training program for adults. Waltham (MA): UpToDate; 2019.

32. American College of Sports Medicine position stand. Progression models in resistance training for healthy adults. Med Sci Sports Exerc 2009;41:687.

33. Li F, Harmer P, Fitzgerald K, et al. Effectiveness of a therapeutic tai ji quan intervention vs a multimodal exercise intervention to prevent falls among older adults at high risk of falling: a randomized clinical trial. JAMA Intern Med 2018;178(10): 1301–10.

34. Li F, Harmer P, Fisher J, et al. Tai chi and fall reductions in older adults: a randomized controlled trial. J Gerontol A Biol Sci Med Sci 2005;60(2):187–94.

35. Wang C, Schmid CH, Iversen MD, et al. Comparative effectiveness of tai chi versus physical therapy for knee osteoarthritis: a randomized trial. Ann Intern Med 2016;165:77–86.

36. Wang C, Schmid CH, Rones R, et al. A randomized trial of tai chi for fibromyalgia. N Engl J Med 2010;363(8):743–54.
37. Wayne PM, Walsh JN, Taylor-Piliae RE, et al. Effect of tai chi on cognitive performance in older adults: systematic review and meta-analysis. J Am Geriatr Soc 2014;62:25–39.
38. Ren X, Li Y, Yang X, et al. The effects of tai chi training in patients with heart failure: a systematic review and meta-analysis. Front Physiol 2017;8:989.
39. Raman G, Zhang Y, Minichiello VJ, et al. Tai chi improves sleep quality in healthy adults and patients with chronic conditions: a systematic review and meta-analysis. J Sleep Disord Ther 2013;2(6):141.
40. Chen KM, Chen MH, Chao HC, et al. Sleep quality, depression state, and health status of older adults after silver yoga exercises: cluster randomized trial. Int J Nurs Stud 2009;46(2):154–63.
41. O'Halloran PD, Blackstock F, Shields N, et al. Motivational interviewing to increase physical activity in people with chronic health conditions: a systematic review and meta-analysis. Clin Rehabil 2014;28(12):1159–71.
42. Morgan K, Tan MP. Behaviour change theories and techniques for promoting physical activity among older people. In: Nyman SR, Barker A, Haines T, et al, editors. The Palgrave handbook of ageing and physical activity promotion. Cham (Switzerland): Springer International Publishing; 2018. p. 211–29.
43. Son NK, Ryu YU, Jeong HW, et al. Comparison of 2 different exercise approaches: tai chi versus Otago, in community-dwelling older women. J Geriatr Phys Ther 2016;39(2):51–7.
44. Buchner DM, Beresford SAA, Larson EB, et al. Effects of physical activity on health status in older adults II: intervention studies. Annu Rev Public Health 1992;13(1):469–88.

Mindfulness, Stress, and Aging

Katarina Friberg Felsted, PhD

KEYWORDS

- Mindfulness • MBSR • Older adults • Chronic conditions

KEY POINTS

- Mindfulness is an effective treatment for a variety of chronic conditions in older adults, because it is simple, inexpensive, and continues to show improvement over time.
- Mindfulness reduces stress and improves mental function in older adults, including cognitive function, anxiety, depression, sleep quality, loneliness, and posttraumatic stress disorder.
- Mindfulness reduces stress and improves physical function, including cardiovascular conditions, diabetes, rheumatoid arthritis, Parkinson disease, urge urinary incontinence, and chronic pain.

INTRODUCTION

As our population seeks to age optimally, the role of stress must be factored into the quest. Chronic stressors decrease the body's ability to recover from stress, creating mental and physical vulnerabilities. Mentally, stresses influence otherwise normative aging in the immune system, and its effects with age are interactive.[1] Physically, chronic stress suppresses both cellular (intracellular pathogens) and humoral (parasites and bacteria) immunity and affects functional measures; the older the age of participants studied, the more pronounced their decreases were.[2,3]

Although mindfulness meditation (MM) has its roots in Buddhism, traced back several thousand years, it has been introduced into scientific circles over the last several decades as a treatment for stress, particularly chronic stress. Modern mindfulness was pioneered in the late 1970s by Dr Jon Kabat-Zinn at the University of Massachusetts Medical School. Mindfulness is defined as paying attention to the present moment in a purposeful, nonjudgmental way. Dr Kabat-Zinn created the Mindfulness-Based Stress Reduction (MBSR) program, an 8-week program with a 2.5-hour session once a week for 8 weeks, with a daylong retreat between weeks 6 and 7.[4] Participants are encouraged to practice their mindfulness through audio recordings and specific

University of Utah College of Nursing, 10 South Connor Road, #3655, Salt Lake City, UT 84112, USA
E-mail address: katarina.felsted@nurs.utah.edu
Twitter: @katarinafelsted (K.F.F.)

Clin Geriatr Med 36 (2020) 685–696
https://doi.org/10.1016/j.cger.2020.06.010
0749-0690/20/© 2020 Elsevier Inc. All rights reserved.

skills they learn in sessions. MBSR is applied to a variety of concerns and does not need to be modified to fit a specific condition.

This program has been modified in a myriad of ways in the last several decades. Another evidence-based MM program, which incorporates mindfulness training as well as cognitive therapy, is Mindfulness-Based Cognitive Therapy (MBCT).[5] MBCT was originally created to treat depression and has been used across other chronic conditions since its inception. Beyond MBSR and MBCT, other versions of MM programs are often referred to simply as mindfulness. Mindfulness programs may and do differ greatly from one another in the way that they are offered: variations in duration, frequency, practice options, location, and ways of transmission. In research it also is applied to a variety of populations: age, race and ethnicity, heterogeneity in physical and mental circumstances. The constant within each mindfulness program, regardless of its adaptations, is that it trains participants in a skill that allows the mind to be "calm, clear, open-hearted, and devoid of suffering."[6] Becoming aware and accepting of the present moment allows participants to respond authentically to their current experience, which is preferable to reflexively letting the mind be reactive and judgmental and which can potentially worsen the person's situation instead.

CONTENT
Why Older Adults Are Excellent Candidates for Mindfulness

Mindfulness and self-compassion have been shown to improve older adults' coping capabilities as well as their adaptation to stressful situations. Recent research has shown that mindfulness may improve resilience and positive reappraisal while reducing anxiety and stress as well as negative self-focus.[7] The research by Sorrell[8] on MM specifically in an older adult population found that mindfulness results in changed brain structure as it is related to stress and memory. As such, she suggests that health care professionals should consider mindfulness as "a helpful intervention for older adults with problems such as depression, anxiety, chronic pain, loneliness, and caregiver burden."

Mindfulness is particularly efficacious for older adults with chronic conditions. Self-management of chronic conditions has much to do with health-related behaviors, because compliance with recommendations has a large effect on how much of the chronic condition is controlled. These conditions include stress, anxiety, and depression as well as cardiovascular disease, diabetes, and more. Mindfulness has been shown to positively affect health-related behaviors in older adult participants and significantly reduce stress.[9,10] Older adults coping with various chronic mental and physical health conditions often present with anxiety. A recent review of 7 randomized controlled trials (RCTs) using mindfulness in a specifically geriatric population supported the use of MBSR and MBCT to reduce geriatric anxiety.[11]

Mindfulness as a buffer between stress and health-related quality of life was examined in a cross-sectional study of community-dwelling healthy older adults. Results identified an inverse relationship between stress and both mental and physical health. de Frias and Whyne[12] suggest that "mindfulness is a powerful, adaptive strategy that may protect older adults from the well-known harmful effects of stress on mental health."

Stress research also indicates that immune function decreases with stress and normal aging. Older adults are prone to late life stressors in the form of loss of spouse or close friends, relocation from independent living, and managing chronic conditions/comorbidities. Stress in older adults may speed the effects aging has on immune system function.[2] Given this link between stress, aging, and the immune system, mindfulness may prove particularly germane for older adults, because it helps reduce emotional reactivity, which occurs through "cognitive and affective mechanisms of action and neural activation of the cingulate cortex, amygdala, and hippocampus."[13]

Other reasons make mindfulness an encouraging course for older adult interventions. Older adults exhibit a higher than usual adherence rate to mindfulness programs. This impressive adherence rate is seen not only during the intervention but also at follow-up, with some follow-up points being at 6 and 12 months.[10,14–16] High adherence may be explained by the fact that older adults have rich life experience to bring to meditation, and being introduced to a "reflective, stationary intervention" could be an engaging modality.[17] As correlation, older adults may be more skilled at effective learning, the concept of how practice helps one respond better and better to a treatment.[18]

Older adults are also a population that may benefit more than younger adults by using an integrative, nonpharmacologic treatment. Age is significantly associated with negative pharmacologic side effects, and these can be more disconcerting in older adults. Furthermore, older adults may have fewer funds available for prescription and nonprescription drugs. Certain medications also show reduced efficacy with time. Given these reasons, using mindfulness to treat chronic conditions in older adults may be an important way to prepare for better health care in the growing older adult population.[19]

Mindfulness Application to Chronic Mental Health Conditions in Older Adults

Cognitive impairment

Several studies examine mindfulness' role in addressing issues related to cognitive impairment in older adults. For example, MBSR has been shown to increase executive function, with significance persistent at a 21-week follow-up.[20] Sustained findings regarding cognitive impairment in older adults are particularly noteworthy, because aging is generally associated with cognitive detriment and cannot be assumed to remain stable.[21,22]

MBSR has shown improved clinical outcomes on memory composite scores in older adults with neurocognitive difficulties in a multisite trial using a health education control condition. At a 3-month follow-up, improvement in worry, depression, and anxiety was evident.[23] As mentioned, MBSR tends to show sustained and even stronger outcomes at later follow-up.

In another study, participants showed improvements in memory, reduced worry severity, and increased mindfulness. The multisite trial offered an elongated 12-session MBSR group, containing the same components and using additional repetition. The extended version (12-week) provided no additional gains with regards to clinical or cognitive outcomes, satisfaction, or continued practice as compared with the 8-week version. These findings indicated that older adults are able to achieve significant improvement using the standardized, manualized 8-week session protocol, and most were continuing to practice at a 6-month follow-up.[24] Researchers noted that a mindfulness intervention may prove to hold a high value in public health, because anxiety and cognitive impairment are often found in the older adult population.

It has been assumed that older adults with more advanced stages of dementia are unable to benefit from mindfulness practices, because they require awareness of the present moment and a capacity to identify and accept one's feelings or reactions. However, a recent study was the first to include older adults in long-term care with dementia ranging from moderate to severe in a mindfulness versus cognitive activity to explore outcomes. Researchers used a crossover design, and "significant short-term changes in agitation, discomfort, anger, and anxiety" were found in the mindfulness group versus the cognitive activity group.[13] Residents in long-term care, as well those providing their care, may benefit from a reduced emotional reactivity in the resident.

Sleep quality

Cognitive daytime impairment has been linked to poor sleep quality. The population with the highest percentage of sleep problems is older adults: more than half of those 55 and older have some type of sleep disturbance, which holds true when assessed with biological measures as well as self-report measures.[25] A RCT with a mindfulness awareness practice and an active sleep hygiene education comparison group showed significantly superior improvements in the mindfulness group compared with the sleep hygiene education group in both biological and self-report measures.[26] Furthermore, improvements in the mindfulness group in sleep-related daytime impairment measures of anxiety, depression, fatigue, and stress were all statistically significant between groups.[26]

A qualitative study by Hubbling and colleagues[27] using MBSR as treatment for chronic insomnia uncovered the 4 following themes: the impact of mindfulness on sleep and motivation to adopt a healthy sleep lifestyle; benefits of mindfulness on aspects of life beyond sleep; challenges and successes in adopting mindfulness-based practices; and the importance of group sharing and support. MBSR proves as effective as prescription sedatives in treating chronic insomnia, but has few or no side effects.[28,29] The bypassing of pharmacologic negative side effects may be even more important in older adults.

A secondary analysis of an MBSR study and associated sleep changes in older adults (65 years and older) showed significant effect sizes in improved sleep.[30] It is notable that higher effect sizes correlated with poorer sleep quality scores at baseline, indicating that those with the worst sleep quality to begin with gained the most improvement. These significant findings remained at 6-month follow-up. A second sleep quality RCT, recruiting older adults (75 and older) with chronic insomnia to participate in an MBSR program, assessing its effectiveness on insomnia as well as combined anxiety or depressive symptoms also found significant effect on both insomnia and depression.[31] It is notable that MBSR was found to be a useful intervention for chronic insomnia, even when the insomnia is combined with anxious or depressive symptoms.

Older adults are more susceptible to depression as a result of stress, and the relationship between sleep quality and depression continues to be strong. A recent pilot study comparing MM with vacation time as a control examined variables related to depression. Participants were aged 55 to 90 years, and mindfulness showed improvements in sleep quality as well as other depression variables, including severity of pain.[32]

Loneliness

Along with sleep difficulties, older adults often experience loneliness in later life. Moving away from an independent living situation, loss of spouse or partner, and mortality affecting friendships and close ties are all potential causes. Researchers have found that loneliness is correlated with an increased proinflammatory gene expression,[33] which in turn may initiate the development and progression of acute and chronic conditions that contribute to comorbidities and mortality.[34] Given this potential cascade, addressing loneliness in older adults holds considerable value.

Prior studies of MBSR have shown its capacity to reduce inflammatory protein biomarkers.[35] A recent trial sought to examine MBSR's effectiveness in reducing loneliness and its concurrent biological threat to health in older adults. As predicted by researchers, a standardized 8-week MBSR program reduced loneliness, whereas it increased in the control group. It also evidenced a reduction of "downregulated NF-κB-associated gene expression profile" as well as C-reactive protein.[33] The downregulation of these 2 gene expressions in the mindfulness group evidenced a reduction in the inflammatory protein, indicating a protective effect on immunity as loneliness decreased. It is noteworthy that loneliness in the control group did not remain the same but worsened and may have been accompanied by exacerbated inflammation as a result.

Posttraumatic stress disorder

Posttraumatic stress disorder (PTSD) is an all too common concern in older adults, with one likely correlation being the veteran older population. According to the Pew Research Center, two-thirds of the veteran population are older adults. Unfortunately, the veteran population often does not receive sufficient PTSD treatment from their primary care provider and continue to suffer from functional impairment, poorer mental and physical health, and higher suicide rates.[36] Possemato and colleagues[37] conducted an RCT using primary care brief mindfulness training, an abbreviated 4-session mindfulness based on MBSR, compared with treatment as usual. Exploratory analyses revealed that "the describing, nonjudging, and acting with awareness facets of mindfulness may account for decreases in PTSD." This conclusion is often drawn from research results, describing why mindfulness is found efficacious and effective with such a variety of conditions.

Patients with subclinical levels of PTSD may still suffer PTSD-like symptoms. Cortisol levels tend to correlate with PTSD symptoms and are thus a useful indicator of PTSD. An RCT using semiweekly mindfulness-based stretching and deep breathing exercise (MBX) against a control group in an 8-week intervention sought to establish whether this type of mindfulness could normalize cortisol levels and thus reduce PTSD symptoms in older adult veterans.[38] Symptoms were measured at baseline, 4 weeks, 8-week completion, and 16-week follow-up. MBX outcomes were superior to the control group severity of symptoms and serum cortisol and were sustained at the 16-week follow-up mark.[38] Again, outcomes of mindfulness training continued to be significant at a follow-up point beyond intervention completion, indicating the persisting efficacy of mindfulness interventions.

A misconception exists that mindfulness may not be a feasible treatment option for a veteran PTSD population, because the focus on the present moment could be psychologically triggering in increased symptoms. However, an MM intervention in a veteran PTSD population found that veterans engaged at a higher level than called for and that no adverse reactions were reported. Furthermore, the MM was statistically significantly superior to the psychoeducational comparison arm in reducing PTSD symptoms in participants, in self-reported as well as clinician-administered measures.[39]

The effects of mindfulness have been studied in other related vulnerable older adult populations. A recent study examined older adult Nigerian Fulani herdsmen, who are often vulnerable to attacks from farmers as the herdsmen move their cattle from 1 spot to another. The role of positive reappraisal was examined within the relationship between mindfulness and well-being. According to researchers' findings, mindfulness interventions are valuable in promoting well-being in later life, because mindfulness was found to be independently associated with "better life satisfaction, lower perceived stress, and fewer depressive symptoms."[40]

Mindfulness Application to Chronic Physical Conditions in Older Adults

Cardiovascular disease

Two-thirds of older adults have hypertension, a risk factor for cardiovascular disease, which is the leading cause of death.[41] For this reason, hypertension is often referred to as the silent killer. Mindfulness interventions to reduce blood pressure have been shown effective in specific comorbid populations of patients with prostate cancer, patients with breast cancer, cancer survivors, and type II diabetics.[42-44] Palta and colleagues[17] examined diastolic and systolic blood pressure in a sample of older adult African Americans with high blood pressure at baseline. Although the social support control group showed increased diastolic blood pressure at intervention completion, statistically significant reductions in both systolic and diastolic blood pressure were shown in the MBSR group. Furthermore, attendance rates were 98%, indicating high acceptability. Because many older adults remain unaware and undiagnosed, mindfulness may be a particularly important treatment for other comorbidities, because it would potentially positively affect conditions the older adult is unaware they have.

Hypertension in a sample of older adult participants with chronic kidney disease (CKD) has also been explored. MM, a brief technique to reduce stress, was tested in CKD patients and compared with an education intervention. Study participants received 3 separate interventions: a 14-minute MM and a 14-minute education session in random order at 2 separate visits. MM resulted in statistically significant reduction in both systolic and diastolic blood pressure, reduced heart rate, and reduced arterial pressure, a striking finding because the entire intervention occurred in less than 15 minutes.[45] A small subset of the participants in the study was given a controlled breathing intervention to determine if the slowed breathing of MM was the mechanism for these significant improvements. No changes in hemodynamics were observed with sole controlled breathing, signifying that the breathing component alone will not alter cardiovascular measures.

Diabetes

Diabetes carries an emotional burden with its management, because the disease can be a harbinger of additional serious comorbidities, such as cardiovascular disease, neuropathy, and kidney disease.[46] Fisher and colleagues[47] estimate that up to 40% of diabetics are subject to emotional distress and impaired well-being. Using cross-sectional data, Son and colleagues[46] examined the relationship of mindfulness with anxious and depressive symptoms in 666 diabetic participants; analyses showed significant associations with mindfulness being inversely proportional with both anxiety and depressive symptoms in people with diabetes. Researchers concluded that mindfulness "shows promise as a potentially protective characteristic against the influence of stressful events on emotional well-being."[46]

A related study sought to explore whether an adapted MBSR training would prove effective in reducing distress and improving diabetes self-efficacy, self-management, and A1C scores. Training included a 90-minute session during an education class on diabetes. Study participants were instructed to perform 10-minute daily home practices over the 3-month study period. Statistically significant improvements were shown in A1C scores, self-management, and self-efficacy as related to diabetes from baseline to 3-month completion.[48] Retention and satisfaction measures also proved feasible and acceptable.

Rheumatoid arthritis

Mindfulness has also been shown to affect both distress and disease activity in rheumatoid arthritis (RA) populations. Two studies have recently demonstrated mindfulness' statistically significant role in reducing psychological distress, not only at study completion but also at 6- and 12-month follow-up.[49,50] Clinician-assessed RA disease activity also demonstrated reductions in stiffness, pain, tender joints, and patient global assessments.[50] No significant findings were found regarding swollen joints or C-reactive protein levels.

Parkinson's disease

Parkinson's disease is the most common movement disorder and the second most common neurodegenerative disease of aging.[51] Current treatment is pharmacologic, and the negative side effects can be severe. According to Advocat and colleagues,[52] this has created a trend to apply holistic approaches that includes mindfulness. As such, their RCT examined mindfulness with a wait-list control group and its effects on both function and well-being. Although changes at completion were not significant, by the 6-month follow-up, both function and well-being had reached statistical significance.[53] These findings underscore the long-term benefits of a mindfulness intervention on Parkinson disease function and well-being.

MBSR has also been examined for its benefits on nonmotor symptoms in Parkinson's patients. Participants received the standard 8-week MBSR course with a 16-week follow-up. Depression levels, anxiety, and stress were all statistically significantly decreased at intervention completion and at the 16-week follow-up.[54]

Urge urinary incontinence

Urge urinary incontinence (UUI) is a chronic condition that affects as many as half of older adult women. Few seek treatment; UUI is either seen as a stigma and too sensitive of a topic to raise with one's primary care provider, or it is assumed to be a normal part of aging. Studies have shown mindfulness may be effective in treating older adult women's UUI, with reduced bother and severity symptoms, as well as a reduction in perceived stress.[14–16] Results for various measures were statistically sustained at diverse intervals, including as long as 1 year.

Chronic pain

Chronic pain is another condition in which nonpharmacologic treatments are becoming more urgent. The original MBSR protocol was created to address chronic pain.[55] Mindfulness is being used to address nonspecific chronic pain, and results are staying significant through the 6-month follow-up, highlighting how mindfulness continues to effectively address conditions long after the participant's intervention.[56]

Low back pain (LBP) treatment in older adults is limited because of the negative side effects of analgesics in this population. Many older adults deal with chronic LBP, and several mindfulness studies have been administered to explore its efficacy. A mindfulness intervention for chronic LBP in older adults improved short-term function as well as long-term pain. The improved function did not remain at follow-up.[57] However, an RCT using MBSR to treat CLBP found reduced pain and improved function, which was sustained at 1-year follow-up and still noted at a 2-year follow-up.[58,59] A qualitative, grounded theory study of MM on older adults with CLBP found MM to result in "less pain, improved attention, better sleep, and enhanced well-being, and improved quality of life."[60]

SUMMARY
Wide Application

Substantial research has shown MM's strong significant results in the treatment of both mental and physical chronic conditions in older adults. It appears to be a simple, elegant tool for meeting complex conditions in the geriatric population and does not dilute when applied to more severe conditions. In fact, research has shown that the more stressed the participant at baseline, the greater the improvement at completion and follow-up.[23] Furthermore, it does not need to be tailored to a specific condition to be effective.

Improvement Across Several Areas

A common result that weaves through these studies on mental and physical conditions often found in older adults is that mindfulness improves many items at once. It is rare to effectively isolate 1 measure and see improvement in only that measure, making it even more valuable as a potential treatment, because multiple chronic conditions and comorbidities are likely to exist in older adulthood. Applications of mindfulness may address high blood pressure and depression at once or may address diabetic symptoms and improve sleep quality at the same time. Large RCTs find support for the uses of MBSR and MBCT specifically with older adults on a wide variety of conditions: chronic LBP, chronic insomnia, improved sleep quality, enhanced positive affect, reduced symptoms of anxiety and depression, and improved memory and executive functioning.[11]

Cost-Effective

Mindfulness is quite inexpensive, because it is learned within 1 course. No refresher classes or skill updates are needed. Medications and other treatments may bring decreased efficacy with time; mindfulness treatment does the exact opposite, with efficacy continuing to increase over time. Furthermore, this capability may allow for less prescription medication to be administered, an important development because medications tend to prove more dangerous in the older adult population, where polypharmacy and contraindications between medications are commonplace.

Future Research

For these reasons, it is crucial that further large-scale trials be conducted. Mindfulness research is a current funding priority of the National Center for Complementary and Integrative Health at the National Institutes of Health.[61] As health care providers work with an increasing aging population, additional mindfulness research is also recommended to study clusters of chronic conditions. Mindfulness may be uniquely suited to address several symptom clusters at once.

DISCLOSURE

The Hartford Center for Geriatric Nursing Excellence Jonas Center for Nursing and Veterans Healthcare Gamma Rho Chapter of Sigma Theta Tau International Office of the Associate Vice President for Health Equity and Inclusion, University of Utah College of Nursing Research Support Grant, University of Utah.

REFERENCES

1. Graham JE, Christian LM, Kiecolt-Glaser JK. Stress, age, and immune function: toward a lifespan approach. J Behav Med 2006;29(4):389–400.
2. Hawkley LC, Cacioppo JT. Stress and the aging immune system. Brain Behav Immun 2004;18(2):114–9.
3. Segerstrom SC, Miller GE. Psychological stress and the human immune system: a meta-analytic study of 30 years of inquiry. Psychol Bull 2004;130(4):601–30.
4. Kabat-Zinn J. Mindfulness-based stress reduction (MBSR). Constructivism in the Human Sciences 2003;8(2):73–107.
5. Segal ZV, Teasdale JD, Williams JMG. Mindfulness-based cognitive therapy: theoretical rationale and empirical status. In: Hayes SC, Follette VM,

Linehan MM, editors. Mindfulness and acceptance: expanding the cognitive-behavioral tradition. New York: Guilford Press; 2004. p. 45–65.

6. Shastri PS. Mindfulness and older adults: reviewing the historical foundations of mindfulness in practice and the development of a mindful meditation program for older adults. Ann Arbor(MI): ProQuest Information & Learning; 2016.

7. Perez-Blasco J, Sales A, Meléndez JC, et al. The effects of mindfulness and self-compassion on improving the capacity to adapt to stress situations in elderly people living in the community. Clin Gerontol 2016;39(2):90–103.

8. Sorrell JM. Meditation for older adults: a new look at an ancient intervention for mental health. J Psychosoc Nurs Ment Health Serv 2015;53(5):15–9.

9. Salmoirago-Blotcher E, Hunsinger M, Morgan L, et al. Mindfulness-based stress reduction and change in health-related behaviors. J Evid Based Complement Altern Med 2013;18(4):243–7.

10. Ribeiro L, Atchley RM, Oken BS. Adherence to practice of mindfulness in novice meditators: practices chosen, amount of time practiced, and long-term effects following a mindfulness-based intervention. Mindfulness (N Y) 2018;9(2):401–11.

11. Greenawalt KE, Orsega-Smith E, Turner JL, et al. The impact of "The Art of Happiness" class on community dwelling older adults: a positive psychology intervention. Act Adapt Aging 2019;43(2):118–32.

12. de Frias CM, Whyne E. Stress on health-related quality of life in older adults: the protective nature of mindfulness. Aging Ment Health 2015;19(3):201–6.

13. Kovach CR, Evans C-R, Sattell L, et al. Feasibility and pilot testing of a mindfulness intervention for frail older adults and individuals with dementia. Res Gerontol Nurs 2018;11(3):137–50.

14. Felsted KF, Supiano KP. Mindfulness-based stress reduction versus a health enhancement program in the treatment of urge urinary incontinence in older adult women: a randomized controlled feasibility study. Res Gerontol Nurs 2019;12(6):285–97.

15. Baker J, Costa D, Guarino JM, et al. Comparison of mindfulness-based stress reduction versus yoga on urinary urge incontinence: a randomized pilot study. With 6-month and 1-year follow-up visits. Female Pelvic Med Reconstr Surg 2014;20(3):141–6.

16. Baker J, Costa D, Nygaard I. Mindfulness-based stress reduction for treatment of urinary urge incontinence: a pilot study. Female Pelvic Med Reconstr Surg 2012;18(1):46–9.

17. Palta P, Page G, Piferi RL, et al. Evaluation of a mindfulness-based intervention program to decrease blood pressure in low-income African-American older adults. J Urban Health 2012;89(2):308–16.

18. Gaylord SA, Palsson OS, Garland EL, et al. Mindfulness training reduces the severity of irritable bowel syndrome in women: results of a randomized controlled trial. Am J Gastroenterol 2011;106(9):1678–88.

19. Rowe JW, Fulmer T, Fried L. Preparing for better health and health care for an aging population. JAMA 2016;316(16):1643–4.

20. Moynihan JA, Chapman BP, Klorman R, et al. Mindfulness-based stress reduction for older adults: effects on executive function, frontal alpha asymmetry and immune function. Neuropsychobiology 2013;68(1):34–43.

21. Aine CJ, Sanfratello L, Adair JC, et al. Development and decline of memory functions in normal, pathological and healthy successful aging. Brain Topogr 2011;24(3–4):323–39.

22. Wang M, Gamo NJ, Yang Y, et al. Neuronal basis of age-related working memory decline. Nature 2011;476(7359):210–3.

23. Wetherell JL, Hershey T, Hickman S, et al. Mindfulness-based stress reduction for older adults with stress disorders and neurocognitive difficulties: a randomized controlled trial. J Clin Psychiatry 2017;78(7):e734–43.

24. Lenze EJ, Hickman S, Hershey T, et al. Mindfulness-based stress reduction for older adults with worry symptoms and co-occurring cognitive dysfunction. Int J Geriatr Psychiatry 2014;29(10):991–1000.

25. Ancoli-Israel S, Ayalon L. Diagnosis and treatment of sleep disorders in older adults. Am J Geriatr Psychiatry 2006;14(2):95–103.

26. Black DS, O'Reilly GA, Olmstead R, et al. Mindfulness meditation and improvement in sleep quality and daytime impairment among older adults with sleep disturbances: a randomized clinical trial. JAMA Intern Med 2015;175(4):494–501.

27. Hubbling A, Reilly-Spong M, Kreitzer MJ, et al. How mindfulness changed my sleep: focus groups with chronic insomnia patients. BMC Complement Altern Med 2014;14:50.

28. Winbush NY, Gross CR, Kreitzer MJ. The effects of mindfulness-based stress reduction on sleep disturbance: a systematic review. Explore (NY) 2007;3(6): 585–91.

29. Bootzin RR, Epstein DR. Understanding and treating insomnia. Annu Rev Clin Psychol 2011;7:435–58.

30. Gallegos AM, Moynihan J, Pigeon WR. A secondary analysis of sleep quality changes in older adults from a randomized trial of an MBSR Program. J Appl Gerontol 2018;37(11):1327–43.

31. Zhang J-X, Liu X-H, Xie X-H, et al. Mindfulness-based stress reduction for chronic insomnia in adults older than 75 years: a randomized, controlled, single-blind clinical trial. Explore (NY) 2015;11(3):180–5.

32. Wahbeh H, Nelson M. iRest meditation for older adults with depression symptoms: a pilot study. Int J Yoga Therap 2019;29(1):9–17.

33. Creswell JD, Irwin MR, Burklund LJ, et al. Mindfulness-Based Stress Reduction training reduces loneliness and pro-inflammatory gene expression in older adults: a small randomized controlled trial. Brain Behav Immun 2012;26(7): 1095–101.

34. Hackett RA, Hamer M, Endrighi R, et al. Loneliness and stress-related inflammatory and neuroendocrine responses in older men and women. Psychoneuroendocrinology 2012;37(11):1801–9.

35. Lengacher CA, Kip KE, Barta MK, et al. A pilot study evaluating the effect of mindfulness-based stress reduction on psychological status, physical status, salivary cortisol, and interleukin-6 among advanced-stage cancer patients and their caregivers. J Holist Nurs 2012;30(3):170–87.

36. Pew Research Center. The changing face of America's veteran population. FAC-TANK 2019. Available at: https://www.pewresearch.org/fact-tank/2017/11/10/the-changing-face-of-americas-veteran-population/. Accessed December 3, 2019.

37. Possemato K, Bergen-Cico D, Treatman S, et al. A randomized clinical trial of primary care brief mindfulness training for veterans with PTSD. J Clin Psychol 2016; 72(3):179–93.

38. Kim SH, Schneider SM, Bevans M, et al. PTSD symptom reduction with mindfulness-based stretching and deep breathing exercise: randomized controlled clinical trial of efficacy. J Clin Endocrinol Metab 2013;98(7):2984–92.

39. Niles BL, Klunk-Gillis J, Ryngala DJ, et al. Comparing mindfulness and psychoeducation treatments for combat-related PTSD using a telehealth approach. Psychol Trauma 2012;4(5):538–47.

40. Aliche JC, Onyishi IE. Mindfulness and wellbeing in older adults' survivors of herdsmen attack the mediating effect of positive reappraisal. Aging Ment Health 2020;24(7):1132–40.

41. Bragg SW. Hypertension in older adults. Ann Longterm Care: Clinical Care and Aging 2015;23(12):42–3.

42. Carlson LE, Speca M, Faris P, et al. One year pre-post intervention follow-up of psychological, immune, endocrine and blood pressure outcomes of mindfulness-based stress reduction (MBSR) in breast and prostate cancer outpatients. Brain Behav Immun 2007;21(8):1038–49.

43. Matchim Y, Armer JM, Stewart BR. Effects of mindfulness-based stress reduction (MBSR) on health among breast cancer survivors. West J Nurs Res 2011;33(8):996–1016.

44. Rosenzweig S, Reibel DK, Greeson JM, et al. Mindfulness-based stress reduction is associated with improved glycemic control in type 2 diabetes mellitus: a pilot study. Altern Ther Health Med 2007;13(5):36–8.

45. Park J, Lyles RH, Bauer-Wu S. Mindfulness meditation lowers muscle sympathetic nerve activity and blood pressure in African-American males with chronic kidney disease. Am J Physiol Regul Integr Comp Physiol 2014;307(1):R93–101.

46. Son J, Nyklíček I, Nefs G, et al. The association between mindfulness and emotional distress in adults with diabetes: could mindfulness serve as a buffer? Results from Diabetes MILES: the Netherlands. J Behav Med 2015;38(2):251–60.

47. Fisher L, Skaff MM, Mullan JT, et al. A longitudinal study of affective and anxiety disorders, depressive affect and diabetes distress in adults with Type 2 diabetes. Diabet Med 2008;25(9):1096–101.

48. DiNardo M, Saba S, Greco CM, et al. A mindful approach to diabetes self-management education and support for veterans. Diabetes Educ 2017;43(6):608–20.

49. Nyklíček I, Hoogwegt F, Westgeest T. Psychological distress across twelve months in patients with rheumatoid arthritis: the role of disease activity, disability, and mindfulness. J Psychosom Res 2015;78(2):162–7.

50. Fogarty FA, Booth RJ, Gamble GD, et al. The effect of mindfulness-based stress reduction on disease activity in people with rheumatoid arthritis: a randomised controlled trial. Ann Rheum Dis 2015;74(2):472–4.

51. Mhyre TR, Boyd JT, Hamill RW, et al. Parkinson's disease. Subcell Biochem 2012;65:389–455.

52. Advocat J, Russell G, Enticott J, et al. The effects of a mindfulness-based lifestyle programme for adults with Parkinson's disease: protocol for a mixed methods, randomised two-group control study. BMJ Open 2013;3(10):e003326.

53. Advocat J, Enticott J, Vandenberg B, et al. The effects of a mindfulness-based lifestyle program for adults with Parkinson's disease: a mixed methods, wait list controlled randomised control study. BMC Neurol 2016;16(1):166.

54. Birtwell K, Dubrow-Marshall L, Dubrow-Marshall R, et al. A mixed methods evaluation of a mindfulness-based stress reduction course for people with Parkinson's disease. Complement Ther Clin Pract 2017;29:220–8.

55. Kabat-Zinn J. An outpatient program in behavioral medicine for chronic pain patients based on the practice of mindfulness meditation: theoretical considerations and preliminary results. Gen Hosp Psychiatry 1982;4(1):33–47.

56. la Cour P, Petersen M. Effects of mindfulness meditation on chronic pain: a randomized controlled trial. Pain Med 2015;16(4):641–52.

57. Morone NE, Greco CM, Moore CG, et al. A mind-body program for older adults with chronic low back pain: a randomized clinical trial. JAMA Intern Med 2016; 176(3):329–37.
58. Cherkin DC, Anderson ML, Sherman KJ, et al. Two-year follow-up of a randomized clinical trial of mindfulness-based stress reduction vs cognitive behavioral therapy or usual care for chronic low back pain. JAMA 2017;317(6):642–4.
59. Cherkin DC, Sherman KJ, Balderson BH, et al. Effect of mindfulness-based stress reduction vs cognitive behavioral therapy or usual care on back pain and functional limitations in adults with chronic low back pain: a randomized clinical trial. JAMA 2016;315(12):1240–9.
60. Morone NE, Lynch CS, Greco CM, et al. I felt like a new person." The effects of mindfulness meditation on older adults with chronic pain: qualitative narrative analysis of diary entries. J Pain 2008;9(9):841–8.
61. US Dept of Health and Human Services. NCCIH's funding priorities and research focus 2017. Modified 9/17/2019. Accessed September 26, 2019.

The Role of Prevention in Healthy Aging

Neema Sharda, MD*, Serena Wong, DO, Heidi White, MD, MHS, MEd

KEYWORDS

- Disease prevention • Disability prevention • Healthy aging

KEY POINTS

- As the population ages, a primarily medical model is inadequate to successfully prevent disease and disability.
- The "Welcome to Medicare" and "Annual Wellness Visits" are prime opportunities to focus on personalized prevention plans that include recommended screenings and immunizations.
- Clinic visits can allow health care teams to target impactful outcomes such as prevention of debility, hospitalization, loss of independence, disease progression, and other geriatrics syndromes.
- The Population Health Model is an evolving strategy for prevention at the population level using system-level support and interprofessional collaboration.

INTRODUCTION

As health care professionals desire to adopt and teach approaches to healthy aging described in previous articles, a medical model that focuses on disease alone becomes inadequate. In the context of aging with all of its heterogeneity, we desire to prevent more than disease and promote more than personal choices that influence health. In the broadest context we want to promote healthful activity that is meaningful and personalized to each individual and supported by the larger context of health care systems and local communities.

As we develop our roles individually and collectively through prevention and promotion, we must recognize the impact of the physiology of aging (for example, reduced renal function, changes in muscle vs adipose tissue, and musculoskeletal alterations) and the consequences of disease, but also the person or population in their environment. We must start with a model that will allow us to consider and manipulate all of the factors that contribute to health and function while minimizing disability. In its

Geriatrics Division, Duke University, Duke University Medical Center, Box 3003, Durham, NC 27710, USA
* Corresponding author.
E-mail address: Neema.Sharda@duke.edu
Twitter: @neekap1234 (N.S.); @serenawongs (S.W.); @heidiwhite10 (H.W.)

Clin Geriatr Med 36 (2020) 697–711
https://doi.org/10.1016/j.cger.2020.06.011
0749-0690/20/© 2020 Elsevier Inc. All rights reserved.

International Classification of Functioning, Disability and Health, the World Health Organization has combined the medical model of disease with a social model of disability.[1] In this biopsychosocial model (**Fig. 1**), the outcome of interest is activity (ie, the execution of a task or action) and can be applied to an individual or population. Activity is influenced simultaneously by disease, body function, and structure (ie, including impairments) and participation, including life situations such as role fulfillment in work and family, and community or leisure activities. Importantly, environmental and personal factors provide a context that influence activity achievement. Extrinsic environmental factors (for example, social attitudes, local culture, and architectural characteristics, as well as climate, food availability, and so forth) should be taken into account. Also, intrinsic personal factors like gender, age, coping styles, social capital, education, experiences, and preferences influence how disability and disease are experienced by the individual.

Using this framework, we can apply prevention and promotion activities to any individual, regardless of their degree of health or well-being. We can acknowledge factors outside the medical model that exert influence. We can evaluate a variety of proposed prevention targets such as debility, hospitalization, loss of independence, progression of disease/frailty, loss of dignity, medication errors, social isolation, and falls/injury.

In this article, we describe practical approaches to disease and disability prevention across the spectrum of function and prognosis encountered among older adults. We highlight opportunities to gather necessary information, target meaningful outcomes, and implement standard recommendations. Finally, we provide a discussion of system-level support and interprofessional collaboration to improve health care access and facilitate older adults' activity within their community of living.

The routine clinic visit is a prime opportunity for individualized prevention of disease and disability in older adults. Admittedly, prevention in older adults can be far more complex; however, through iterative monitoring and evaluation, protocols can be devised to create a successful, person-centered approach. As we aim to prevent

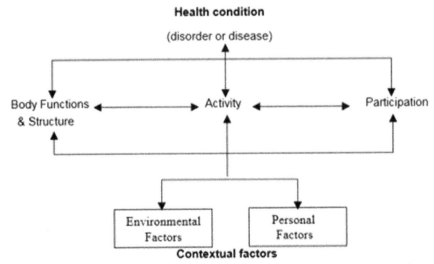

Fig. 1. Interactions between the components of ICF (International Classification of Functioning) (WHO 2001:18). (*Reprinted from* World Health Organization. Towards a common language for functioning, disability and health. International Classification of Functioning, Disability and Health. 2002:1-22.)

disease and disability, we not only consider primary prevention, but secondary, and tertiary prevention as well, known as "Leavell's Levels." Primary prevention is prevention of a disease or disability, for example, through administration of immunizations. Secondary prevention involves early identification of asymptomatic disease, for example, by mammography or bone scan. Finally, tertiary prevention indicates management of symptomatic disease to prevent complications.[2] For example, diabetic patients routinely undergo foot examinations, which may lead to recommendations of therapeutic shoes or self-management training. The US Preventive Services Task Force makes several screening recommendations (**Table 1**); these include screening for depression, diabetes, falls, osteoporosis, and heart disease. In addition, patients born between 1945 to 1965 are eligible for hepatitis C screenings. Cancer screenings include breast, colorectal, and lung.[3,4]

OPPORTUNITIES IN "WELCOME TO MEDICARE" AND "ANNUAL WELLNESS VISITS"

Although prevention begins at birth, the "Welcome to Medicare" preventive visit is a one-time appointment to promote general health and prevent diseases. This visit may be the first time patients review their ability to function safely in their home and community with their providers. Subsequently, the "Medicare Annual Wellness Visit" is the yearly appointment with one's primary care provider to update the personalized prevention plan based on individual health and risk factors. Health risk assessments are commonly used to better understand the patient's health status (including vision, hearing, skin, and dental care), injury risks, behavioral risks, and urgent health needs. This visit is also imperative to gain an understanding of who comprises the patient's interprofessional and caregiver team, which is critical knowledge for when crises arise; for example, in addition to their primary care provider, patients may regularly see and trust their cardiologist, nephrologist, gastroenterologist, and/or endocrinologist. Some older adults have used caregivers and others may rely on community resources, neighborhood friends, or family near and far.[4] Wellness visits are an optimal opportunity to address preventive care; however, given time constraints and the complex needs of many older adults, providers may need to consider more frequent office visits.

Encouraging a healthy lifestyle is the cornerstone of disease and disability prevention. The American Heart Association (AHA) and the American College of Sports Medicine (ACSM) provide exercise recommendations for adults older than 65 years, including aerobics, muscle strengthening, flexibility, and balance. Recognizing that engagement in these programs can feel overwhelming to patients, the AHA and ACSM recommend a stepwise introduction to physical activity to improve safety and adherence.[5] The benefits of exercise include, but are not limited to, reducing cardiovascular disease risk, reducing the risk of dementia and depression, reducing the risk of falls and fall-related injuries, and improving quality of life.[6,7] The National Institute on Aging also provides resources on healthy aging for older adults; these include a focus on (1) exercise, (2) maintaining a healthy weight, (3) healthy eating habits, and (4) participating in enjoyable activities.[8] In addition, local Area Agencies on Aging support free evidence-based disease prevention and health promotion programs, such as on chronic disease self-management and "A Matter of Balance."[9] Finally, Medicare supports the well-known "Silver Sneakers" program, which offers fitness classes designed for seniors at no additional cost.[10]

Immunizations are a key pillar in disease prevention. Given concerns of immune senescence, or declining immune function with age, particular attention should be paid to vaccinating "younger" older adults as advised.[11] The Advisory Council for Immunization Practices (ACIP) of the Centers for Disease Control and Prevention (CDC)

Table 1
US Preventive Services Task Force (USPSTF) A and B recommendations

Topic	Description	Grade	Release Date of Current Recommendation
Abdominal aortic aneurysm: men	The USPSTF recommends 1-time screening for abdominal aortic aneurysm by ultrasonography in men ages 65–75 y who have ever smoked.	B	June 2014
Alcohol misuse: screening and counseling	The USPSTF recommends that clinicians screen adults age 18 y or older for alcohol misuse and provide persons engaged in risky or hazardous drinking with brief behavioral counseling interventions to reduce alcohol misuse.	B	May 2013
Blood pressure screening: adults	The USPSTF recommends screening for high blood pressure in adults aged 18 y or older. The USPSTF recommends obtaining measurements outside of the clinical setting for diagnostic confirmation before starting treatment.	A	October 2015
Breast cancer screening	The USPSTF recommends screening mammography for women, with or without clinical breast examination, every 1–2 y for women age 40 y and older.	B	September 2002
Colorectal cancer screening	The USPSTF recommends screening for colorectal cancer starting at age 50 y and continuing until age 75 y.	A	June 2016
Depression screening: adults	The USPSTF recommends screening for depression in the general adult population. Screening should be implemented with adequate systems in place to ensure accurate diagnosis, effective treatment, and appropriate follow-up.	B	January 2016
Diabetes screening	The USPSTF recommends screening for abnormal blood glucose as part of cardiovascular risk assessment in adults aged 40–70 y who are overweight or obese. Clinicians should offer or refer patients with abnormal blood glucose to intensive behavioral counseling interventions to promote a healthful diet and physical activity.	B	October 2015
Falls prevention: older adults	The USPSTF recommends exercise interventions to prevent falls in community-dwelling adults 65 y or older who are at increased risk for falls.	B	April 2018

Hepatitis C virus infection screening: adults	The USPSTF recommends screening for hepatitis C virus (HCV) infection in persons at high risk for infection. The USPSTF also recommends offering 1-time screening for HCV infection to adults born between 1945 and 1965.	B	June 2013
Lung cancer screening	The USPSTF recommends annual screening for lung cancer with low-dose computed tomography in adults ages 55–80 y who have a 30 pack-year smoking history and currently smoke or have quit within the past 15 y. Screening should be discontinued once a person has not smoked for 15 y or develops a health problem that substantially limits life expectancy or the ability or willingness to have curative lung surgery.	B	December 2013
Osteoporosis screening: women	The USPSTF recommends screening for osteoporosis in women age 65 y and older and in younger women whose fracture risk is equal to or greater than that of a 65-year-old white woman who has no additional risk factors.	B	January 2012
Statin preventive medication: adults ages 40–75 y with no history of cardiovascular disease (CVD), 1 or more CVD risk factors, and a calculated 10-y CVD event risk of 10% or greater	The USPSTF recommends that adults without a history of CVD (ie, symptomatic coronary artery disease or ischemic stroke) use a low- to moderate-dose statin for the prevention of CVD events and mortality when all of the following criteria are met: (1) they are ages 40–75 y; (2) they have 1 or more CVD risk factors (ie, dyslipidemia, diabetes, hypertension, or smoking); and (3) they have a calculated 10-y risk of a cardiovascular event of 10% or greater. Identification of dyslipidemia and calculation of 10-y CVD event risk requires universal lipids screening in adults ages 40–75 y.	B	November 2016

From U.S. Preventive Services Task Force. USPSTF A and B recommendations. 2018. Available at: https://www.uspreventiveservicestaskforce.org/Page/Name/uspstf-a-and-b-recommendations/; with permission.

recommends a vaccine schedule (**Table 2**).[12] There have been extensive public health efforts to increase vaccination rates. In 2014, the ACIP recommended a routine use of a series of pneumococcal vaccines in adults ≥65 years old; the aim was to prevent 230 cases of invasive pneumococcal disease and 12,000 cases of community-acquired pneumonia over the lifetime of a single cohort of persons aged 65 years in the United States.[13] Despite efforts to improve vaccination rates, the CDC reports that in 2016 to 2017, only 60% of Medicare beneficiaries had claims data for receiving at least 1 pneumococcal vaccine. It is noteworthy that implementation of pneumococcal vaccine recommendations has not been equal across all older adults. White beneficiaries have disproportionately higher claims data for these vaccines; differences may be attributed to attitudes toward vaccines and concern about vaccination safety. In addition, beneficiaries with chronic or immunosuppressive medical conditions were more likely to be vaccinated.[14] The American Medical Association has recognized challenges to improving immunization rates and has recommended 4 steps to overcome these challenges: (1) make vaccination easy by offering convenient hours and walk-in appointments; (2) offer encouragement through anecdotes and remind patients about those who cannot be vaccinated, such as infants; (3) leverage the patient-provider relationship: the provider can send jargon-free recommendations directly to the patient regarding the importance of immunizations; and (4) the health care team should work together to track and monitor vaccination completion.[15] Finally, the CDC provides "Vaccine Information Statements"; these are information sheets that explain the benefits and risks of vaccines. Federal law mandates that these are provided to patients, and also serve as an opportunity for patient education.[16]

TARGETING IMPACTFUL OUTCOMES

Screenings for substance abuse are another component of the Annual Wellness Visit. Data suggest that from 2005 to 2014, binge alcohol use and alcohol use disorders significantly increased among older adults.[17,18] This is concerning because as adults age, several physiologic changes occur, including (1) the liver enzymes that metabolize alcohol become less efficient, (2) the central nervous system becomes more sensitive to the effects of alcohol, and (3) a decrease in lean body mass increases the effective concentration of alcohol. In addition, older adults who misuse alcohol are at increased risk of medication interactions, depression, memory problems, and sleep disturbances.[18] Notably, more than a tenth of older adults in the United States are estimated to be binge drinkers; literature suggests that binge drinkers also have higher

Table 2	
Recommended immunizations by the Centers for Disease Control and Prevention for adults ≥65 years	
Influenza	1 dose annually
Tdap or Td	1 dose Tdap then Td booster every 10 y
Varicella	2 doses (4–8 wk apart)
Zoster	2 doses of recombinant zoster vaccine (2–6 mo apart, age ≥50) or 1 dose of zoster vaccine live
Pneumococcal (PCV 13)	1 dose
Pneumococcal (PPSV 23)	1 dose

Data from Centers for Disease Control and Prevention. Recommended immunization schedule for adults aged 19 years or older, United States, 2018.

concurrent tobacco use.[19] Many older adults may be unaware that recommended alcohol limits are lower with increasing age, and prevention may include education about age-appropriate recommendations. One validated screening instrument that is, commonly used is the Alcohol Use Disorders Identification Test (AUDIT); this is a 10-item questionnaire that can then trigger clarifying questions. The literature suggests that brief interventions in a variety of health care settings may be impactful to reduce drinking; however, there are few systematic studies of alcohol treatment outcomes in older adults.[18]

The independence of older adults can be threatened by several events, including falls and hospitalizations. For example, the consequences of falls include, but are not limited to, head injury, fracture, decreased mobility, loss of independence with activities of daily living, and decreased quality of life. At the annual wellness visit, providers have the opportunity to collect relevant data: screen for hearing impairment, take an inventory of durable medical equipment that the patient owns, complete a thorough review of medications and indications, and screen for cognitive impairment. The CDC has established the STEADI (STopping Elderly Accidents, Deaths and Injuries) Initiative to help providers prevent falls in community-dwelling older adults. This includes the following: (1) identifying patients as low, moderate, or high risk for a fall; (2) identifying modifiable risk factors; and (3) offering effective interventions. Modifiable risk factors that lend to intervention include gait and balance problems, vitamin D deficiency, vision impairment, foot ailments, and polypharmacy.[20,21] The framework for prevention in older adults also includes deprescribing. This may involve transitioning to nonpharmacological interventions for insomnia, anxiety, stress, and pain management to avoid adverse drug reactions and interactions, which are sources of iatrogenic disability and decline for older adults. In addition, the Canadian Deprescribing Network offers resources for deprescribing to patients and health care professionals, such as educational videos, algorithms, and handouts.[22] When considering hospitalizations, primary care providers or specialists such as geriatricians or cardiologists often learn if a patient plans an elective procedure. This can be a critical time to educate patients and their families on preventing dangers of hospitalization, such as adverse drug events, delirium, malnutrition, and infection.[23,24]

Although the Medicare Annual Wellness Visit helps guide our treatment plan for the year, the complex balance of resilience and frailty in older adults who are phenotypically varied can be challenging. Screening to prevent disease and disease complications is a multifaceted decision. The University of California San Francisco created an online tool (eprognosis.ucsf.edu) to help the clinician objectively consider prognosis to help with decision making. This tool is a compilation of validated indices, and the clinician can apply it to patients living at home, in a nursing facility, in the hospital, or enrolled with hospice.[25] In addition, geriatricians at Saint Louis University have outlined outpatient clinical glidepaths; this is a valuable approach that allows clinicians to consider health management in the context of life expectancy and degree of dependence. Each procedure, as outlined in **Table 3**, provides a recommendation based on 4 categories: (1) robust elderly, life expectancy ≥5 years and functionally independent; (2) frail, life expectancy less than 5 years or significant functional impairment; (3) moderate dementia, life expectancy 2 to 10 years; and (4) end of life, life expectancy less than 2 years.[26]

POPULATION HEALTH MANAGEMENT: A MODEL FOR PREVENTION

Traditionally, medical providers have taken a disease-specific approach to health, focusing on diagnoses like heart disease, diabetes, hypertension, cancer, and so

Table 3
The health maintenance clinical glidepath

Procedure	Robust Elderly Life Expectancy ≥5 Years and Functionally Independent	Frail Life Expectancy <5 Years or Significant Functional Impairment	Moderate Dementia Life Expectancy 2–10 Years	End of Life Life Expectancy <2 Years
Office visits	Do once a year	Do 1–4 times/y	Do 1–4 times/y	Do as needed
blood pressure including orthostatics	Do each visit	Do each visit	Do each visit	Do each visit
Weight	Do each visit; if loss of >5 lb/y, perform Mini Nutritional Assessment	Do each visit; if loss of >5 lb/y, perform Mini Nutritional Assessment	Do each visit; if loss of >5 lb/y, perform Mini Nutritional Assessment	Don't do
Height	Do once a year	Do once a year	Don't do	Don't do
Cholesterol screening	Consider screening for patients aged 65–75 if additional risk factors (eg, smoking, diabetes mellitus, hypertension)	Consider screening for patients aged 65–75 if additional risk factors (eg, smoking, diabetes mellitus, hypertension)	Don't do	Don't do
Breast examination	Do yearly	Do yearly	Do yearly	Don't do
Mammography	Do every 1–2 y up to age 80	Consider every 1–2 y up to age 75	Consider every 1–2 y up to age 70	Don't do
Papanicolaou (Pap) smear	Consider 1–3 Pap smears if patient has never had	Don't do	Don't do	Don't do
Prostate specific antigen	Discuss pros and cons with patient	Discuss pros and cons with patient	Discuss pros and cons with caregiver	Don't do
Fecal occult blood test	Do yearly	Consider yearly	Consider yearly	Don't do
Colonoscopy	Consider every 5 y	Don't do	Don't do	Don't do
Influenza vaccine	Do yearly	Do yearly	Do yearly	Do yearly
Pneumococcal vaccine	Do once; consider repeat every 6 y for patients with chronic disease	Do once	Do once	Consider vaccination once

Tetanus	Do primary series if not vaccinated before and booster every 10 y	Do primary series if not vaccinated before	Do primary series of not vaccinated before	Don't do
Thyroid stimulating hormone	Do every 2 y	Do every 2 y	Do every 3 y	Consider
Lifestyle education (exercise, smoking cessation, alcohol, and injury prevention)	Do every visit	Do every visit	Discuss periodically with caregiver	Don't do
Aspirin	Do, if history of myocardial infarction or ≥2 cardiovascular risk factors	Do, if history of myocardial infarction or ≥2 cardiovascular risk factors	Do, if history of myocardial infarction or ≥2 cardiovascular risk factors	Don't do
Men: Ask about erectile dysfunction and androgen deficiency in aging men screen for hypogonadism	Do yearly	Do yearly	Consider yearly	Don't do
Visual acuity testing	Consider every year	Consider every year	Consider every year	Don't do
Hearing impairment	Consider every year	Consider every year	Consider every year	Don't do
Ask about urinary incontinence	Do yearly	Do yearly	Do yearly	Do yearly
Maintain awareness of elder abuse	Do each visit	Do each visit	Do each visit	Do each visit
Assess activities of daily living (ADLs) and instrumental ADLs	Do yearly	Do each visit	Do each visit	Do each visit
Fasting blood glucose	Do, if symptomatic or 3 y if has risk factors	Do, if symptomatic or 3 y if has risk factors	Do, if symptomatic or 3 y if has risk factors	Consider if symptomatic
Cognitive screening	Do initially; do if symptomatic	Do initially; do if symptomatic	Do initially	Consider if symptomatic

(continued on next page)

Table 3
(continued)

Procedure	Robust Elderly Life Expectancy ≥5 Years and Functionally Independent	Frail Life Expectance <5 Years or Significant Functional Impairment	Moderate Dementia Life Expectancy 2–10 Years	End of Life Life Expectancy <2 Years
Depression screening	Do initially; do if symptomatic	Do initially; do if symptomatic	Do initially; do if symptomatic	Do initially; do if symptomatic
Screening for gait and balance	Do initially; do if symptomatic	Do initially; do if symptomatic	Do initially; do if symptomatic	Do if symptomatic
Sleep apnea	Do yearly	Do yearly	Do each visit	Don't do
Pain assessment	Do each visit	Do each visit	Do each visit	Do each visit
Medication review including over-the-counter and herbal medications	Do each visit	Do each visit	Do each visit	Do each visit
Osteoporosis	Do at least once; consider at 2-y intervals	Do at least once	Do at least once	Don't do
Advance directives	Do yearly and as needed	Do yearly and as needed	Do yearly and as needed	Do yearly and as needed

From Flaherty JH, Morley JE, Murphy DJ, et al. The development of outpatient Clinical Glidepaths. J Am Geriatr Soc. 2002;50(11):1886–1901; with permission.

forth. As people age, however, many accumulate comorbidities, and it becomes progressively more complex to adequately address their health needs. The concept of population health management (PHM) developed in the early 2000s as a way to improve the health of people in a population. PHM programs have 3 basic goals, also known as the "Triple Aim": (1) to improve health, (2) improve the health care experience, and (3) to reduce health care costs.[27] PHM focuses on a much broader scope than simply the diagnosis and treatment of a patient's illnesses. Instead, it assesses the relationships of different factors that influence the health of members of a population over their life course, and applies this knowledge in practice and policy to improve the health of the population.[28]

PHM systems incorporate information from sources including risk assessments, surveys, health records, and claims data to analyze the population's risks and to guide targeted health improvement initiatives.[29] Considerations of PHM programs and research include individual medical care, public health policies and interventions, social determinants of health, environment, and healthy behaviors. PHM programs work to analyze population-based factors, use these data to risk stratify patients, and create patient-centered interventions to reduce disease progression and improve quality of life.[30] Generally, population health strategies are holistically focused on physical functioning, psychological well-being, social well-being, and self-rated successful aging[31] and may partner with community resources to improve health education and access (**Table 4**). Lifestyle behavior interventions, such as increased physical activity, healthier diet, and decreased usage of tobacco products, are often part of PHM programs. These interventions usually require frequent contact with patients and a multimodal approach (such as in person, telephone, and online), tailored to the population being served.

One example of a PHM model is the accountable care organization (ACO), a Medicare program created under the Affordable Care Act in 2010. The term ACO describes a group of providers who take responsibility for the health of a group of people. Designed to address the Triple Aim of improved quality, reduced costs, and increased satisfaction, ACOs are value-driven models of care focused on improving the health of the population of people attributed to their care.[32] One example is a hospital system whose designated population is the Medicare patients who live within their catchment area. In this example, Medicare assigns patients to an ACO on a yearly basis, based on their previous claims data. The ACO receives financial incentives to reduce health care costs for their population of patients, motivating it to find ways to improve quality preventive care and reduce complications due to chronic disease.[33] Some ACOs have partnered with community resources to improve social determinants of health within their geographic region. For example, the Cincinnati Children's Hospital Medical Center has helped fund community health initiatives partnering with local organizations to address preventable health factors such as accidental injuries, uncontrolled asthma, and poor nutrition. One project involved evaluating medical records of people with multiple admissions for asthma; using neighborhood mapping, analysts were able to identify substandard housing units owned by the same landlord. With the help of a local legal aid group, they were able to influence the landlord to make improvements to the housing.[33]

Medicare Advantage Organizations (MAOs) are also engaging in PHM approaches to deliver value-based care. MAOs promote wellness including tobacco cessation and discounts for exercise and nutrition. They monitor population risks and assess psychosocial needs to provide targeted health education and care management to high-risk patients or those with chronic conditions. For frail older adults, MAOs can provide services including increasing transportation for community services and to

Table 4
Examples of population health management strategies

Area of Focus	Examples of Population Health Management Strategies
Disease prevention	• Increase access to recommended immunizations and screening for high-risk conditions • Enable lifestyle modification programs and incentivize healthy behaviors • Analyze claims data and neighborhood statistics to identify risks specific to the target population, such as environmental exposures and access to healthy food • Identify behavioral risk factors using reports from local police departments and school districts
Chronic disease management	• Use health coaches to educate people about their diseases and how to avoid complications • Create shared decision-making tools • Design patient tools for improved care plan adherence • Evaluate pharmacy data to track likelihood of hospitalization • Build patient engagement through motivational coaching, addressing health literacy, and teaching skills for improved patient self-management • Use case management and care coordination interventions, including mobilization of a multidisciplinary team to support high-quality care, facilitation of communication between providers and patients, help with medication management, and monitor transitions of care
Social determinants of health	• Improve access to transportation • Establish support for those with inadequate finances • Community support for smoking cessation and healthy meal preparation • Internet-use training for older adults to reduce loneliness and risk of victimization and fraud

Data from Jain S, Wilk A, Thorpe K, et al. A model for delivering population health across the care continuum. Am J Accountable Care. 2018;9(3):16-22; and Tkatch R, Musich S, MacLeod S, et al. Population health management for older adults: review of interventions for promoting successful aging across the health continuum. Gerontol Geriatr Med. 2016;2:2333721416667877.

address social isolation; care management; home safety assessments and in-home visits; and medication management alerts.[34]

Another example of a PHM model is the Geriatric Resources for Assessment and Care of Elders (GRACE) model of care, which targets low-income older adults.[35] In this program, the GRACE support team (including a nurse practitioner, geriatrician, social worker, pharmacist, physical therapist, mental health social worker, and community-based services liaison) performs a comprehensive geriatric assessment and develops a personalized care plan to address geriatric syndromes. The team partners with the primary care provider to implement a patient-centered plan, using a longitudinal tracking system to monitor progress. Enrolled patients have the benefit of their support team helping them navigate the health system across different providers and sites of care, improving continuity, and reinforcing patient-centered goals.

Some PHM models focus on a specific disease, selecting patients with that disease as their population (such as heart failure or diabetes). These disease-based programs may mostly emphasize the medical perspective, whereas PHM programs with a broader scope may help emphasize the important psychosocial factors that affect health. An exception to this are PHM programs designed to address dementia care.

Created at the Durham Veterans Affairs Medical Center, one example is the Caring for Older Adults and Caregivers at Home (COACH) program.[36] This program uses an interprofessional team to assess and support older adults with dementia and their family caregivers. A social worker and nurse perform home visits to assess safety gaps, medication compliance, caregiver burden, and dementia symptoms. Cases are reviewed with a broader team including a geriatrician, geriatric psychiatrist, and geriatric pharmacist, and care plans are communicated with primary care providers. Depending on need, follow-up is performed by phone or home visit. Goals include supporting function and home safety, supporting and educating caregivers, and reducing institutionalization. Because of pilot program success, COACH is being expanded regionally to more rural areas. However, more funding and legislative support are needed to develop dementia-specific PHM programs nationwide. Especially in the older population, where there tend to be an accumulation of chronic disease and increasingly complex social situations, an important area of focus in public policy will be how to best design and implement PHM systems to benefit aging adults.

SUMMARY

Health care professionals are adopting a biopsychosocial approach to understanding potential targets to promote healthy aging for both individuals and communities. Each of us has opportunities to collect relevant data for the purpose of formulating individualized prevention and health promotion plans. These plans should take into consideration prognosis, disability, and life expectancy. PHM allows health care professionals to collaborate to address barriers to health care access, target populations at risk, and address environmental contributors to health and well-being.

DISCLOSURE

The authors have nothing to disclose.

REFERENCES

1. World Health Organization. Towards a common language for functioning, disability and health. International Classfication of Functioning, Disability and Health. Geneva (Switzerland): World Health Organization; 2002. p. 1–22.
2. Katz DL, Elmore JG, Wild DMJ. Jekel's epidemiology, biostatistics, preventive medicine, and public health [electronic resource]. Philadelphia: Saunders; 2014.
3. U.S. Preventive Services Task Force. USPSTF A and B recommendations. 2018. Available at: https://www.uspreventiveservicestaskforce.org/Page/Name/uspstf-a-and-b-recommendations/.
4. Welcome to Medicare preventive visit. 2019. Available at: www.medicareinteractive.org. Accessed October 29, 2019.
5. Nelson ME, Jack Rejeski W, Blair SN, et al. Physical activity and public health in older adults: recommendation from the American College of Sports Medicine and the American Heart Association. Circulation 2007;116(9):1094–105.
6. Morey M. Physical activity and exercise in older adults. UpToDate; 2019.
7. de Souto Barreto P, Rolland Y, Vellas B, et al. Association of long-term exercise training with risk of falls, fractures, hospitalizations, and mortality in older adults: a systematic review and meta-analysis. JAMA Intern Med 2019;179(3):394–405.
8. What do we know about healthy aging? 2018. 2019. Available at: https://www.nia.nih.gov/health/what-do-we-know-about-healthy-aging. Accessed December 6, 2019.

9. Healthy aging. 2019. 2019. Available at: https://www.n4a.org/healthyaging. Accessed December 6, 2019.

10. Silver Sneakers. 2019. Available at: https://www.silversneakers.com/. Accessed December 6, 2019.

11. High K. Immunizations in older adults. Clin Geriatr Med 2007;23(3):669–85.

12. Centers for Disease Control and Prevention. Recommended immunization schedule for adults aged 19 years or older, United States. Atlanta (GA): Centers for Disease control and prevention; 2018.

13. Tomczyk S, Bennett NM, Stoecker C, et al. Use of 13-valent pneumococcal conjugate vaccine and 23-valent pneumococcal polysaccharide vaccine among adults aged >/=65 years: recommendations of the Advisory Committee on Immunization Practices (ACIP). MMWR Morb Mortal Wkly Rep 2014;63(37):822–5.

14. Black CW, W, Warnock R, et al. Pneumococcal vaccination among US medicare beneficiaries aged >65 years, 2009-2017. 2018. Available at: https://www.cdc.gov/vaccines/imz-managers/coverage/adultvaxview/pubs-resources/pcv13-medicare-beneficiaries.html. Accessed October 25, 2019.

15. Berg S. How to get patients on board with immunization. 2018. Available at: https://www.ama-assn.org/delivering-care/public-health/how-get-patients-board-immunization. Accessed December 17, 2019.

16. Vaccine information Statements. 2019. 2019. Available at: https://www.cdc.gov/vaccines/hcp/vis/index.html. Accessed December 6, 2019.

17. Han BH, Moore AA, Sherman S, et al. Demographic trends of binge alcohol use and alcohol use disorders among older adults in the United States, 2005–2014. Drug Alcohol Depend 2017;170:198–207.

18. Barry KL, Blow FC. Drinking over the lifespan: focus on older adults. Alcohol Res 2016;38(1):115–20.

19. Han BH, Moore AA, Ferris R, et al. Binge drinking among older adults in the United States, 2015 to 2017. J Am Geriatr Soc 2019;67(10):2139–44.

20. Stevens JA. The STEADI tool kit: a fall prevention resource for health care providers. IHS Prim Care Provid 2013;39(9):162–6.

21. Karani MV, Haddad Y, Lee R. The role of pharmacists in preventing falls among America's Older Adults. Front Public Health 2016;4:250.

22. Do I still need this medication? 2017. 2019. Available at: https://www.deprescribingnetwork.ca/. Accessed December 6, 2019.

23. Kresevic DM. Reducing functional decline in hospitalized older adults: learn how to detect and prevent hidden dangers of hospitalization for these patients. Am Nurse Today 2015;10:S8.

24. McDonald SR, Heflin MT, Whitson HE, et al. Association of integrated care coordination with postsurgical outcomes in high-risk older adults: the perioperative optimization of senior health (POSH) initiative. JAMA Surg 2018;153(5):454–62.

25. Lee SS, Alex; Widera, Eric; Yourman, Lindsey; Schonberg, Mara; Ahalt, Cyrus. ePrognosis. Available at: https://eprognosis.ucsf.edu/index.php. Accessed July 1, 2020.

26. Flaherty JH, Morley JE, Murphy DJ, et al. The development of outpatient clinical glidepaths. J Am Geriatr Soc 2002;50(11):1886–901.

27. Berwick DM, Nolan TW, Whittington J. The triple aim: care, health, and cost. Health Aff (Millwood) 2008;27(3):759–69.

28. Guerin S, Stefanacci RG. The psychology behind population health management. Popul Health Manag 2018;21(5):344–5.

29. Jain S, Wilk A, Thorpe K, et al. A model for delivering population health across the care continuum. Am J Accountable Care 2018;9(3):16–22.

30. Cramm JM, Nieboer AP. Is "disease management" the answer to our problems? No! Population health management and (disease) prevention require "management of overall well-being. BMC Health Serv Res 2016;16(1):500.

31. Tkatch R, Musich S, MacLeod S, et al. Population health management for older adults: review of interventions for promoting successful aging across the health continuum. Gerontol Geriatr Med 2016;2. 2333721416667877.

32. Devore S, Champion RW. Driving population health through accountable care organizations. Health Aff (Millwood) 2011;30(1):41–50.

33. Casalino LP, Erb N, Joshi MS, et al. Accountable care organizations and population health organizations. J Health Polit Policy Law 2015;40(4):821–37.

34. Tompkins C, Higgins A, Perloff J, et al. Population health management in Medicare advantage. Health Affairs Blog 2013. https://doi.org/10.1377/hblog20130402.029363. Available at: https://www.healthaffairs.org/do/10.1377/hblog20130402.029363/full/.

35. Counsell SR, Callahan CM, Buttar AB, et al. Geriatric resources for assessment and care of elders (GRACE): a new model of primary care for low-income seniors. J Am Geriatr Soc 2006;54(7):1136–41.

36. D'Souza MF, Davagnino J, Hastings SN, et al. Preliminary data from the Caring for Older Adults and Caregivers at Home (COACH) program: a care coordination program for home-based dementia care and caregiver support in a Veterans Affairs Medical Center. J Am Geriatr Soc 2015;63(6):1203–8.

Best Practices for Promoting Healthy Aging

Kathryn M. Daniel, PhD, RN, AGPCNP-BC, GS-C

KEYWORDS

- Healthy aging • Best practices • Maximum health span

KEY POINTS

- In key communities around the world, some are known for residents who have longer and more vigorous lives with less chronic disease.
- This article summarizes the factors that are common in those communities and how other communities are seeking to adopt some of the factors to benefit more communities—specifically, the blue zones, Experience Corps, and the age-friendly movement.
- The General Ecological model derived from Bronfenbrenner's work and synthesized by Juster best explains this phenomena.
- An active lifestyle, healthy nutrition, and supportive family and cultural group seem to be common across all healthy communities.

This article discusses best practices for promoting healthy aging. As the previous chapters in this issue illustrate, there are many variables that contribute to healthy aging. Many of the best understood contributions to healthy aging involve lifestyle choices across the life span, such as nutrition, physical activity, and social engagement. Best practices involve applying what is known from rigorous scientific investigations and incorporating information learned from large naturally occurring phenomena to recommendations for lifestyle and health management decisions alike. Because aging occurs across a lifetime, rigorous investigation of potential interventions almost always will be limited. Specifically, this article discusses the blue zones, Experience Corps, and the age-friendly movement.

Understanding the rationale for what it is thought to explain the relationships between the variables of environment, lifestyle, diet, culture, and family and the desired outcome of healthy aging leads to a theoretic model of explanation. The model that best describes the relationships between an individual and best practices for healthy aging is derived from Bronfenbrenner's general ecological model.[1] Although Bronfenbrenner used the term, *maximum health span*, for the purposes of this article, that is considered a synonym for healthy aging. Health span is that part of life with limited morbidity and maximum autonomy. It can be described as the years of life that are

College of Nursing and Health Innovation, University of Texas at Arlington, 411 South Nedderman, Box 19407, Arlington, TX 76013, USA
E-mail address: kdaniel@uta.edu
Twitter: @kathydaniel4 (K.M.D.)

Clin Geriatr Med 36 (2020) 713–718
https://doi.org/10.1016/j.cger.2020.06.012
0749-0690/20/© 2020 Elsevier Inc. All rights reserved.

lived independently with little impact by chronic disease while free of pain and disability. The goal is to have maximum health span, which is not the same thing as maximum life span.

There are macrosystem factors, mesosystem factors, microsystem factors, and individual factors that interrelate and explain resilience and the impact on potential for maximal health span (**Fig. 1**). At the individual level, lifestyle choices further expand or contract an individual's resilience. Because some of these factors often are not able to be manipulated, rigorous evidence to support the model is in short supply, but naturally observed phenomena do support the model. Because aging is a process that begins even before birth and is a longitudinal process in humans, observational and population-based studies are the norm and interventional studies are, if not impossible, at the least exceptionally rare. Some of the best known and developed best practices are outlined in this article.

BLUE ZONES

The best evidence to support healthy aging practices comes from observational data from communities around the world, where the desired outcome of extended health

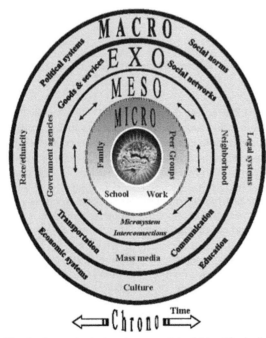

Identified Allostatic Load Factors

Macrosystem
- **Socioeconomics:** education, income, occupational status, downward mobility
- **Race/ethnicity:** Nonwhite
- **Spirituality:** religious attendance, sense of meaning/purpose

Exosystem
- **Neighborhoods:** crowding, noise, lack of housing, rural/urban
- **Social networks:** emotional support, ties with friends/neighbours, social position

Microsystem
- **Family:** attachment, violence/turmoil, single parent, separation, care-giving, demands/criticisms, spouse
- **Work:** control, demands, decisions, career instability, effort-reward imbalance
- **Peer groups:** homelessness/squatter

Individual
- **Genetics:** ACE rs4968591 gene
- **Personality:** type A/hostility, locus of control

Fig. 1. An ecological systems model of identified allostatic load antecedents. The central propositions of Bronfenbrenner's general ecological model is that individuals are developmentally shaped by complex reciprocally interacting systems. These interdependent forces consist of the individual's immediate environment (microsystem), the interconnections among several individuals (mesosystems), the indirect influence of social structures and settings (exosystem), and finally the current overarching cultural and subcultural patterns (macrosystem) over time (chronosystem). Examples are provided in the diagram to the left, with parallel risk and protective factors identified in relation to allostatic load listed on the right. (*From* Juster R, McEwen BS, Lupien SJ. Allostatic load biomarkers of chronic stress and impact on health and cognition. Neurosci Biobehav Rev. 2010;35(1):14; with permission.)

span with limited morbidity is observed. Buettner[2] originally identified the blue zones in 2005 as 5 areas around the world in which the population live extraordinarily long and illness-free lives. This initial photojournalism publication in *National Geographic* led to a book in 2008.[3] Common to all these communities is that they are geographically located in temperate climates, that natives eat a wide variety of fruits and vegetables that are locally grown, and that natives live fairly simple, less industrialized lives. All the communities are close to the sea and incorporate fish as part of their diets. Daily activity is a part of everyday life—not vigorous aerobic activity but walking to and from the store and to church and other social and everyday events. The lifestyles are less sedentary than most Americans. The communities are highly socially integrated with intergenerational families that live together.

In 2016, Buettner and Skemp[4] summarized the recommendations of a multidisciplinary team that looked closely at the characteristics of these communities with exceptional aging. They call their recommendations the "Power 9." These recommendations are believed to contribute to slowing the aging process and can be seen in the Bronfenbrenner model.[1] They are as follows:

1. Move naturally. The residents in all these communities did not depend on using motor vehicles or other machines in their daily lives. They were active in their daily lives walking to and from all activities. They frequently cultivated gardens and continued to tend to domesticated animals.
2. Purpose. The residents of these communities did not retire from life once they reached advanced age. They continued to have a purpose in life that directs their daily activities and role in the community. They continued to participate and be engaged in their churches and communities.
3. Downshift. Residents of these long-lived communities practiced daily meditation or prayer that helped them manage the stress in their lives.
4. The 80% rule. Residents of many of these communities learned to stop eating when they are 80% full. Furthermore, they ate their largest meal at midday and only a small meal in the evening; then, it usually was 12 hours to 14 hours before eating again the next day.
5. Plant slant. Their diets were composed predominantly of fruits and vegetables with only a small proportion of animal proteins. The average amount of meat was only 5 servings per month.
6. Wine at 5 pm. Many consumed a modest amount of wine every day (1–2 glasses) with family and friends.
7. Belong. Almost every centenarian in the study was part of a faith-based community and regularly attended worship in their community.
8. Loved ones first. Older adults were part of intergenerational families who all lived together. Parents and grandparents did not move to other accommodations as they aged; they remained in the home amidst the larger family. Divorce was rare; spouses made lifetime commitments to their partners and families, which were honored.
9. Right tribe. Residents often had a close set of friends whom they treasured and celebrated with all their lives. It is hypothesized that this close-knit set of friends served as an accountability resource as well as warding off loneliness and depression.

As a result of these observations, other communities have sought to incorporate the diet, lifestyle, and social conditions of blue zones whenever possible into their own communities so that they too might benefit. Even though the luxury of living in a temperate and sunny latitude may contribute to the outcomes in blue zones and not be accessible by everyone around the world, others can adopt the lifestyles and diet as well as social integration that seem to be just as important.

The adoption of more physical activity in everyday life has been well documented to be associated with more robust vitality. Gentle, everyday, regular physical activity has many benefits and few downsides. Other best practices that also are associated with positive outcomes include balance and stretching activities, such as yoga or tai chi. Activities like climbing stairs every day and walking to and from activities or shopping are valuable. See the Elizabeth Eckstrom's article, "Physical Activity and Healthy Aging," in this issue and others for more details on physical activity.

The promotion of the Mediterranean diet, with its emphasis on plant-based foods and proportionally smaller animal proteins, seems to be common across all blue zones. Some fish is included in all blue zone dietary patterns. Red wine consumed in very modest amounts is associated with greater health span than no wine at all. See the Marissa Black and Megan Bowman's article, "Nutrition and Healthy Aging," in this issue for more details on this topic.

Integration into the community at all ages is important. Being a contributing and vibrant member of the society in which they live not only preserves the social network of older adults but also enables those older adults to make significant contributions to their communities because of their wisdom and experience. Having purpose in life, even at advanced age, is important in the preservation of quality of life and health. The social network around and relationships between community members become ever more important with age. In blue zone communities, older adults remain home with intergenerational families and are respected and contributing members of those families. See the Halina Kusz and Ali Ahmad's article, "Preserving Engagement, Nurturing Resilience," in this issue for more details on this topic.

EXPERIENCE CORPS

The Experience Corps is currently a program initiative of the American Association of Retired Persons (AARP).[5] It connects teachers, schools, and older adults within a community in meaningful exchanges that benefit each participant in unique ways. it provides students with mentoring and skill building. It provides schools with support for teachers and principals and volunteers for program efforts. It provides older adults with meaningful opportunities for both physical and mental growth in their local community. Information about this novel program, initially started in Berkeley, California, in 1997, led to multiple replication efforts and ultimately adoption by AARP as a nationwide effort.[6]

Today there are opportunities for older adults to volunteer in their community's high-need elementary schools in more than 20 cities serving over 30,000 children through this program. There is documented evidence of benefit to the children and to the older adults who participate.[5]

THE AGE-FRIENDLY MOVEMENT

The World Health Organization (WHO) first proposed the ideas around healthy communities in 2015 in their *World Report on Ageing and Health*.[7] They identified 5 key domains that are essential for older adults to maintain their functional abilities. The 5 key domains of functional ability considered essential are for older adults to

- Meet their basic needs
- Learn, grow, and make decisions
- Be mobile

- Build and maintain relationships
- Contribute

These abilities are essential for healthy aging. They allow older adults to be contributing members of their communities, to live safely, to have purpose and value. At the same time, when these abilities are in place, older adults have the potential to experience maximum health span.

How well communities are able to adopt and foster these domains is related to 3 major considerations: (1) older adults must fit their environment; there must be a person-fit; (2) the negative attitudes toward aging that are pervasive and still deeply engrained in social mores must change; those attitudes limit the potential of older adults in almost every way; and (3) the effects of environments influence individuals differently based on an individual's gender, ethnicity, or level of education.

The WHO recommends that each community enhance functional ability in 2 essential ways:

1. Building and maintaining intrinsic capacity, by reducing risks (such as high levels of air pollution), encouraging healthy behaviors (such as physical activity) or removing barriers to them (for example, high crime rates or dangerous traffic), or by providing services that foster capacity (such as health care)
2. Enabling greater functional ability — in other words, by filling the gaps between what people can do given their level of capacity and what they could do in an enabling environment (for example, by providing appropriate assistive technologies or providing accessible public transport or developing safer neighborhoods). In doing these things, it is important to acknowledge that although population-level interventions may improve environments for many older people, many are not able to benefit fully without individually tailored supports.10 (p160)

The first and most basic domain or ability is that of meeting basic needs. This includes the ability to afford and obtain an adequate diet, clothing, housing, health care, and long-term care supports and services. When societies do not ensure that all members of their society have sufficient resources to meet the basic needs of all of the members of their community, then all other domains are threatened. The built environment in communities and the social fabric of communities have an impact on not only the older adult members but also every member of the communities.

These principles have been applied across the globe. In the United States, the AARP has championed the movement across the country and have developed the Liveable Communities Initiative.[8] Basically, becoming an age-friendly community means that the community conducts a self-study looking for barriers and hazards to healthy aging in a community through the built environment of schools, health care, transportation, access to transportation, and exercise. After the self-study, the community develops an action plan to address the issues they face and ultimately applies for recognition as an age-friendly city and to be part of the age-friendly network. The 8 domains of livability that are community features identified by AARP are

1. Outdoor spaces and buildings
2. Transportation
3. Housing
4. Social participation
5. Respect and social inclusion
6. Civic participation and employment
7. Communication and information
8. Community and health services

As a result of age-friendly efforts, now there is more awareness at the community level of how organizations, such as businesses, health care institutions and hospitals as well as even universities, also can earn the status of age-friendly. In every situation, the status of being age-friendly means that the organization acknowledges the wealth of knowledge and experience that older adults can bring to their organization and makes meaningful efforts to involve older adults in every aspect of the organization. As part of the growing awareness of the challenges faced by many older adults in their communities and other organizations, the organizations almost always adopt new ways of thinking and inclusiveness that benefit the whole community. For example, in a community with limited public transportation options, the growing awareness of need for transportation options for older adults who no longer drive or have access to an automobile leads to more transportation options for everyone in the community, not only the older adults. Becoming age-friendly is sustainable, benefits every member of the community, and is a best practice.

In summary, there are many examples and opportunities for implementation of best practices for healthy aging throughout the world. At the core, changing ageist attitudes toward aging and older adults is key to success in every scenario. Older adults represent a growing valuable resource that communities and institutions have the opportunity to appreciate and engage with, so that the whole community benefits because everyone participates in healthy aging.

DISCLOSURE

The author has nothing to disclose.

REFERENCES

1. Juster R, McEwen BS, Lupien SJ. Allostatic load biomarkers of chronic stress and impact on health and cognition. Neurosci Biobehav Rev 2010;35(1):2–16.
2. Buettner D. The secrets of living longer. Natl Geogr 2005;11:2–21.
3. Buettner D. The blue zones: lessons for living longer from the people who've lived the longest. Washington, DC: National Geographic; 2008.
4. Buettner D, Skemp S. Blue zones: lessons from the world's longest lived. Am J Lifestyle Med 2016;10(5):318–21. Available at: https://search.ebscohost.com/login.aspx?direct=true&db=cmedm&AN=30202288&site=ehost-live.
5. Experience corps: our impact. AARP.org Web site. Available at: https://www.aarp.org/experience-corps/our-impact/experience-corps-research-studies/. Accessed January 3, 2020.
6. Fried LP, Freedman M, Endres TE, et al. Building communities that promote successful aging. West J Med 1997;167(4):216–9. Available at: https://search.ebscohost.com/login.aspx?direct=true&db=cmedm&AN=9348750&site=ehost-live.
7. World Health Organization. World report on ageing and health 2015. World Health Organization. Geneva (Switzerland).
8. Liveable communities. AARP liveable communities web site. Available at: https://www.aarp.org/livable-communities/about/. Accessed January 3, 2020.

Getting from Here to There
Motivational Interviewing and Other
Techniques to Promote Healthy Aging

Liana Lianov, MD, MPH*

KEYWORDS

- Motivational interviewing • Health behavior • Health coaching • Positive psychology
- Self-management • Appreciative inquiry

KEY POINTS

- Motivational interviewing, cognitive behavioral restructuring, and positive psychology techniques are key approaches for facilitating health behavior in all adults, including older adults.
- Authentic, autonomous decision making and positive goals are essential factors in achieving health behavior change.
- The health care team can role model effective change strategies (such as SMART goals) and help patients build self-efficacy and health literacy for long-term self-management.
- Potential issues must be addressed when coaching older adults, such as declining cognitive functioning, long-term health habits, and social isolation.
- By applying effective techniques and leveraging needed support, older adults can make changes, and may even have greater capacity to maintain new habits than young adults.

INTRODUCTION

Preventing and treating chronic diseases and improving well-being depend on individual patients' change in lifestyle behaviors. Behaviors are influenced at multiple levels: individual motivation; support from the health team and influential peers; community norms; policies at the institutions where individuals work, volunteer, and learn; and policies at the local, state, and national levels regulating behaviors, such as smoking. Although acknowledging this complex multilayered influence on behavior, this article focuses on the clinical approach in health care settings.

Facilitating behavior change effectively in clinical practice requires cooperation among the patient, the primary medical practitioners, and the health team.[1] These relationships, even in brief clinical encounters, are essential for success. Clinical settings may not always have health coaches, but can involve the health team to implement brief coaching techniques. The latter involves partnering with patients to facilitate

HealthType LLC, Fair Oaks, CA, USA
* PO Box 1461, Fair Oaks, CA 95628.
E-mail address: act@lianalianovmd.com

Clin Geriatr Med 36 (2020) 719–732
https://doi.org/10.1016/j.cger.2020.06.013
0749-0690/20/© 2020 Elsevier Inc. All rights reserved.

self-discovery for advancing self-directed goals, offering education, and serving as a source of accountability. The basic steps of coaching might actually be more effective in older adults, as evidence suggest that aging individuals are generally more conscientious.[2,3]

Major health behavior change techniques essential in coaching include the following:

1. Assessing readiness to change, with a focus on the level of importance of making the change and the confidence level
2. Motivational interviewing
3. Cognitive behavioral techniques
4. The 5 A's: assess, agree, advise, assist, and arrange[4] or emphasis on ask, advise, and act, as the 3 A's[5]
5. Appreciative inquiry
6. Positive psychology techniques

Applying positive psychology techniques as the foundation for all health coaching is highly encouraged to propel the individual to action.

Some positive psychology techniques include envisioning a positive future, leveraging personal strengths to tap into intrinsic motivation and applying the PERMA model of flourishing[6] (defined later in this article) to connect intrinsically satisfying activities with health-related behaviors. The positive psychology approach might be more critical in individuals as they age, because their core motivators tend to shift from managing family and career to maintaining emotional well-being and social relationships,[7] and, in fact older adults are able to manage psychological well-being better than younger populations[8,9] Older individuals have a distinct set of motives than in early phases of life,[10–12] including emotional satisfaction, that can allow them to be more successful at making change.[13] Hence, motivational techniques can leverage psychological resources in the elderly, such as adaptation through various developmental stages and life challenges. Successful experience with deferring immediate gratification to achieve long-term goals is one example.[7]

Special considerations when assisting health behavior change in the elderly include (1) ensuring that they do not have cognitive deficits, memory decline, or sensory deficits (especially in hearing and vision) that might interfere with initiating change strategies and behavior plans,[13–15] and (2) reframing positive future visioning toward short-term goals. Working with caregivers is essential when deficits are identified. In some cases, even without such deficits, individuals with entrenched lifelong habits might have difficulty making changes.[16] On the other hand, although older adults may be more challenged to initiate a new behavior or change an existing one, they may have an easier time maintaining a healthy behavior once achieved.[13]

ESSENTIAL ELEMENTS OF EFFECTIVE HEALTH COACHING

Health behavior coaching often relies on a patient-centered approach to work toward goals set by the patient. Self-discovery, active learning, and experimentation (instead of receiving advice) can inspire change. Coaches encourage self-driven action plans and accountability, providing education and support along the way. This goal-driven process involves the following:

- Helping patients identify desired outcomes
- Setting specific SMART—specific, measurable, achievable, relevant, and time-bound—goals[17]

- Developing step-by-step action plans
- Building self-efficacy through success at small early steps
- Identifying resources and support
- Monitoring progress
- Adjusting action plans based on that progress
- Establishing a plan for follow-up[18,19]

The most used health behavior change theories and models emphasize certain patient attributes for successful change,[20–22] especially the patient's autonomy. The models also highlight the need for flexibility in the behavior change process and goals, developing easy-to-reach short-term goals along the way to long-term goals to build self-efficacy, and addressing solutions for potential problems and barriers to action plans.[5] Moreover, successful behavior change coaching ensures that the plan aligns with the patient's interest and personality (such as preference for a set vs flexible schedule),[23] encourages use of imagery to concretely visualize making change, and leverages a network of support by mates, adult children, friends, and caregivers.[5] The individual's beliefs and expectations about the outcomes resulting from the change, level of optimism, and self-efficacy are key.[1]

Health coaching that involves these elements has been shown to be effective in improving a spectrum of behaviors,[24,25] including healthful eating, physical activity, and adherence to medications.[26–28] Successful outcomes include weight loss[29–32]; lowering blood pressure, lipid levels,[28,33] blood glucose, and hemoglobin A1c[33–36]; and improving overall health status of patients with chronic conditions.[37]

In addition to ensuring the use of key counseling elements, health coaches have traditionally used responses that align with the individual's readiness to change, as well as motivational interviewing and cognitive behavioral techniques, to facilitate forward movement. A new and increasingly adopted approach leverages positive psychology.[38] However, additional research is needed to identify the specific approaches that can be most effective in diverse populations, including aging groups.[39]

MATCHING INTERVENTIONS TO CHANGE READINESS

The stages-of-change or transtheoretical model of behavior change presents a framework with several stages. A person can get stuck, go back and forth, or completely relapse, requiring renewed efforts to change.[40] Offering interventions matched to the patient's stage may enhance the chance for successfully facilitating their progress from one stage to the next with the goal of inciting and sustaining intrinsic motivation for the intended behaviors.[5] **Table 1** shows the stages of change and suggested stage-matched interventions.

HEALTH MOTIVES OF OLDER ADULTS AND THEIR CAPACITY TO MAKE CHANGE

Many aging individuals are able to maintain autonomy, motivation, behavioral self-regulation, and the energy level to pursue their health-related goals.[15] Personal health behavior motives vary across the lifespan with body-related (eg, weight loss), fitness, and stress management motives being more important in middle age. Health motives appear to have greater impact on behaviors as people age. However, as people age, disease symptoms and manifestations may interfere with capacity to do some health behaviors, such as exercise.[41] Also self-regulation may degrade with aging of the brain.[13]

Table 1
Stage-matched interventions[5]

Stage of Change	Stage-Matched Intervention
Precontemplation (not ready to make a change)	Check confidence and importance of making the change. Explore the general benefits of making the change. If this intervention does not work, honor patient's lack of readiness and revisit the issue at a later time.
Contemplation (thinking about making a change)	Discuss the pros and cons of making vs not making the change. Link the anticipated results with current medical condition, the aging process and specific late life goals. Use motivational interviewing.
Preparation (ready, but has not begun or has not achieved the change at the desired level)	Set an action plan with specific steps and a timeline that are realistic and which the patient is confident they can achieve. Address potential barriers, for example, physical, financial, embarrassment. Reframe self-talk to support the change, such as "I'm too old" into "I'm always learning." Focus on short-term benefits of a sense of vitality. Adjust the plan based on progress to ensure success.
Action (making the change at the desired level)	Once the behavior is achieved, facilitate ongoing self-talk and social support for accountability to sustain the behavior.
Maintaining the change	Build a relapse prevention plan for times when the behavior may lapse during travel/vacations or illness. Ensure continued social support.

MULTIPLE LEVELS OF INFLUENCE ON HEALTH BEHAVIORS

Several levels of influence outside of the clinical encounter impact the likelihood of behavior change. On the intrapersonal level, autonomy is important[42]; the individual must not feel coerced and tends to be driven toward competence and achievement,[42] when guided toward authentic, internally motivated goals. Also, self-efficacy, the individual's confidence level in their skills and capacity to accomplish a self-selected goal, can predict success in making a variety of lifestyle changes.[43] Multiple other internal factors influence an individual's actions and can vary over time, even for the same behavior goal.

On the interpersonal and community levels, social support, as well as support from the clinical team/health coach, can assist the individual to persist and address barriers and the potential stress of making change.[44] An individual's behavioral choices are influenced by social and environmental conditions in the family and larger community.[21,42] Patients who have a greater level of readiness to make a change (ie, feel a greater sense of the importance of making the change and greater self-efficacy to make that change) need less support than individuals who experience fewer of these attributes.[22,45] Community and social engagement are especially important as individuals age.[15] Often even just a single important social connection can make a difference in well-being and adherence to health behaviors.[46] However, with the increase in social isolation in the United States, ensuring appropriate social connection and support is a crucial step in successful behavior change.[15]

The clinician and health care team are important interpersonal behavioral change influencers, especially through authentic, empathetic connection with the patient. Nonjudgmental understanding of the patient's perspective helps avoid resistance to behavior change advice, by emphasizing the patient's role in determining the best way to move forward.[41,47] This construct is at the heart of effective counseling communication and represents the core of motivational interviewing[48] (see the section on the provider-patient relationship, later in this article).

HEALTH BEHAVIOR CHANGE TOOLS

Phone, video, and digital communications can improve behavioral outcomes, especially because they can provide more intensive counseling, more frequent touch-points, and can offer the means for personalizing the counseling interventions. Success has been reported in several behavioral areas, such as smoking cessation and healthy nutrition, and has been shown to benefit a variety of populations, including low-income populations. Seniors tend to use older digital technology, such as desktops, and are less likely to use wearable devices and home assistants. Moreover, they are less likely than young adults to use technology to manage their health.[49]

THE ROLE OF MEMORY AND HEALTH LITERACY IN BEHAVIOR CHANGE

Memory storage is important in building new healthy behaviors as ongoing habits. Older adults may be challenged with memory retention to build and maintain health habits due to cognitive function disorders. However, even those without cognitive disorders experience age-related memory storage challenges (relying more on the hippocampus used for short-term memory rather than the prefrontal cortex than in younger individuals).

This type of memory storage is impacted by disruption of non–rapid eye movement slow-wave activity during aging.[50] Hence, assistance with improving sleep may be an additional consideration when coaching older adults to make changes in other health behaviors. Fortunately, the neuroplasticity of the brain allows different parts of the brain to take over tasks that are governed by areas of the brain that have been damaged through stroke, for example,[1] and other medical conditions that are more likely in older adults with years of unhealthy behaviors.

In addition to helping to ensure adequate sleep, the coach can assist the patient to identify health behavior approaches that boost positive emotions and pair the behavior with what is meaningful to the patient. The association of high levels of emotion can help with memory retention,[1] as well as with unconscious drivers of behavior (discussed in more detail in the positive psychology section later in this article). Other practical memory-retention tips can be incorporated into the behavior change coaching interactions with older adults who are learning new skills required for health behavior change. Examples include speaking slowly, avoiding medical jargon, giving minimal information at any one time, show "how-to" pictures and videos, encouraging the patient to take notes, and using the "teach back" method for the patient to show their understanding.[5]

THE ROLE OF THE PROVIDER-PATIENT RELATIONSHIP IN THE CHANGE PROCESS

Rapport in the provider-patient relationship is a crucial element in facilitating behavior change. Empathy through verbal and nonverbal communication demonstrates that the patient is understood and valued, conveying a level of support for making change. Actions that convey empathy (eg, open posture, good eye contact, and nodding) can be taught and medical practitioners who convey empathy can impact health outcomes.[1] One study showed that patients with diabetes who rated their physicians as empathetic were more likely to have lower hemoglobin levels than those who did not.[51] However, in a recent study, this effect was not replicated.[52] A number of nuanced factors may influence the success of provider-patient relationships to enhance their patients' outcomes. Although further study is needed to sort out those factors of success, medical practitioners are encouraged to leverage the power of authentic human connection during clinical encounters.

At the root of coaching is building a foundation for change through authentic and trusted relationships between the coach and the patient. The successful coach needs to honor the patient as the expert with regard to their personal needs and lifestyles and approach the patient with the open attitude that the individual has the desire for well-being and the capacity for change. The medical practitioner/coach role is to facilitate, guide, and empower individuals to realize their "best self," regardless of the age of the patient.

MOTIVATIONAL INTERVIEWING

Motivational interviewing (MI) is an effective evidence-based approach to overcoming the ambivalence that keeps many people from making desired changes in their lives. This technique builds motivation and strengthens commitment to change, responding to resistance, enhancing the patient's confidence, and recognizing readiness to change.[53] The success of MI is based on the spirit of a collaborative approach, rather than specific steps.

The key MI elements include partnership, compassion, evocation, and acceptance through bolstering a sense of self-worth, affirmation, autonomy support, and accurate empathy.[54] Often these elements are framed as honoring the patient's lack of readiness, rolling with resistance to change, and nonjudgmentally bringing to light discrepancies between the current situation (ie, the patient's current behavior and the limitations that those behaviors perpetuate) and the individual's desired future (ie, health and well-being status and the types of activities and life goals that the new health status support).

When a patient rates confidence and importance levels, the coach can ask why the level is that high, initiating a discussion on the reasons for the change being important or the reasons the patient feels confident they can achieve the change. Of course, if the rating is low, this line of questioning should not be used.[55]

MI has been shown to be a highly effective counseling strategy, particularly when combined with cognitive behavioral techniques (CBTs) discussed later in this article.[39] MI can be helpful when the patient is in the early stages of change, especially contemplation, when the patient is considering making the change. Thirty years of evidence has shown the efficacy of MI across a variety of conditions[54] and risk factors with 10% to 20% improvements.[56]

APPRECIATIVE INQUIRY

Another counseling approach useful in health behavior change is appreciative inquiry, which entails a systematic questioning to draw out the best in patients.[57] The goal is to help patients to search for the good in the current situation and then build on that when framing a goal. This approach starts from a powerful place that can build self-efficacy and motivation. The 5 steps of the appreciative inquiry spiral model of development include[57,58] the following:

- Defining: Questions to understand the patient and where the patient is in the health behavior change process, with a focus on what is already working well.
- Discovery: Questions that further explore what the patient feels good about and appreciates within themselves, as well as in their environment/life situation.
- Dream: Questions to draw out the specific, concrete vision of what might occur in a positive future, driving a sense of motivation and hope about making that vision a reality.
- Designing: Questions to outline a process and co-create a specific plan for making changes in current behaviors to move toward the ultimate dream. The more positive the process is, the more likely that the change will be sustained.
- Delivery/Destiny: Questions to review progress with the action plan, highlighting what has gone well, and with a growth mindset, concretely redesigning action areas that need adjustment for future success.

COGNITIVE BEHAVIORAL TECHNIQUES

CBTs are another essential set of techniques for successful health coaching. These techniques teach the patient to become aware of self-talk that may be a hindrance to making change, and to reframe self-talk in realistic, but more helpful ways. The technique helps the patient's capacity to support oneself, especially when faced with behavioral decisions and behavioral challenges.[59]

Studies support using combination of behavioral theory and cognitive behavioral theory to assist patients with dietary habit changes for weight management and improving cardiovascular and diabetes risk factors. Evidence is particularly strong in patients with type 2 diabetes who receive intensive, intermediate (6–12 months), and long-term (>12 months) duration CBT. Such counseling can prevent or delay onset of type 2 diabetes and hypertension.[39]

THE 5 A'S TECHNIQUE

A commonly taught counseling technique, the 5 A's, offers a helpful framework for facilitating behavior change.[4]

- Assess:
  - Ask about behavioral health risk factors that influence behavior change goals.
  - Also ask about the patient's readiness to make the specific change(s).
- Advise:
  - Give clear, concise, specific, and personalized behavior change advice, including the personal health harms and benefits that impact the patient's health condition,[46,60] and tie the advice to patient concerns or circumstances.[61]
  - Adjust advice to account for the individual's level of health literacy.[62]
  - For patients who are not ready to make a change, the process may stop here. The clinician might ask patients whether they agree to recheck readiness at a later time.
- Agree:
  - Collaborate with the patient to help them select appropriate goals based on the treatment plan, the patient's interest in and willingness to change the behavior.

- o A high level of patient involvement fosters the patient autonomy needed for successful change[63] leading to a realistic action plan based on patient's interests and values.[64]
- o This step can set the stage for ongoing active collaboration to monitor and adjust the plan as needed to sustain the behavior.[65]
- Assist:
  - o Use behavior change techniques (eg, CBTs and positive psychology) to guide the patient to build the skills, confidence and social supports necessary to achieve and maintain the action goals.
  - o Other techniques during this step include modeling and rehearsing the desired behavior, self-contracts with self-rewards, increasing behavioral triggers, and training to manage stress that can trigger unhealthy behaviors or spur lapses.[66]
- Arrange:
  - o Routine follow-up is needed through repeat visits, telephone calls, texts, digital app check-ins, or other contact is necessary to ensure accountability, provide support, adjust the plan, and make necessary referrals to resources and intensive counseling.
  - o After the behavior is achieved, follow-up can offer support to ensure maintenance[67] and to develop relapse prevention plans.[68]

POSITIVE PSYCHOLOGY TECHNIQUES FOR HEALTH BEHAVIOR COACHING

Positive psychology science leverages the power of positive emotions and personal strengths.[69] Some techniques include positive future visioning, leveraging individual strengths, and connecting health behaviors to satisfying activities.

Positive Future Visioning

Individuals can envision positive futures that drive them to turn that vision into reality.[70] Action is fueled by hope, optimistic approaches to finding solutions, and realizing that the individual has the power to make change.[71] Framing the vision based on the type of person one wants to be or the things one wants to achieve can activate positive emotions that motivate and sustain personal change.[72] For example, this approach shifts the focus from health behavioral goals, such as weight loss or tobacco cessation, which remind individuals of their inadequacies, to a focus on how the change enhances their lives, for example, feeling well enough to play with their grandkids. **Box 1** lists questions that can prompt this positive future visioning as a driver of change.

Leveraging Individual Strengths

Individuals can also apply individual strengths toward achieving behavioral change. A variety of contexts of strengths have been identified.[71] One framework of personal strengths often used in positive psychology is the 24 character strengths in 6 domains[73]:

1. Wisdom: creativity, curiosity, judgment, love of learning, perspective
2. Courage: bravery, perseverance, honesty, zest
3. Humanity: love, kindness, social intelligence
4. Teamwork: justice, fairness, leadership
5. Temperance: forgiveness, humility, prudence, self-regulation
6. Transcendence: appreciation of beauty and excellence, gratitude, hope, humor, spirituality

---

Box 1
Tips for envisioning a positive future

- "The What": Ask powerful questions that connect health-related goals to a positive future vision. Ask what the patient will be thinking, feeling, and doing when they achieve the goal. What would this change allow the patient to do differently?

- "The How": Ask what small steps can be achieved that over time lead to sustainable change. Sometimes, focusing only on the first step avoids the change process from being overwhelming. What is a single, small thing can you do now to move you toward that positive future? Identify people to support the individual in making the change and brainstorm ways to overcome potential barriers.

- Checking progress toward the positive future vision, in addition to monitoring behavioral progress, is essential to sustaining motivation. For example, logging minutes being physically active is important; but logging how long they can keep up with their grandchildren or garden might be more important.

Individuals can identify their strengths with the Values-in-Action online survey online at no charge.[74] Other strengths surveys and frameworks, and even informal explorations of what the patient sees as their strengths, can be used. Questions about past achievements, praises from family and friends, and activities that feel energizing can help elucidate their strengths. The main aim is for patients to plan how to use these strengths to make progress toward their health behavior goals. This process is more effective than working toward goals without use of strengths,[69] including health behavior goals.[71] For example, some patients might use their strengths in responsibility to stick to a healthy eating plan. Others might use their organizational skills to convene an exercise group.

Connecting Health Behaviors to Positive and Satisfying Activities

The PERMA framework of the 5 main positive psychology-based pillars of flourishing, identified by Martin Seligman,[6] can be leveraged in the service of initiating and sustaining behavior change. These pillars are *positive emotion* resulting from activities that incite positive feelings; *engagement* in activities that lead to a sense of flow, that is, losing track of time; *relationships* and strong social connections; *meaningful* activities that provide a sense of purpose; and *accomplishment* of personal and professional goals. Connecting these types of activities with health behaviors can be more motivating than simply working toward health goals.

Positive emotions are particularly powerful when experienced during health-related behaviors, because they drive unconscious motivation to continue those behaviors. Research on the upward spiral of lifestyle change finds that people who experience positive emotions while engaging in health-related behaviors can navigate their behavioral choices in ways that support future engagement in those behaviors[75] and in maintaining them.[75,76]

All elements of PERMA can be used in the service of promoting and sustaining health behavior change. In addition to positive emotions, engagement and purpose can drive motivation.[71] The pillars of PERMA are interrelated,[77] so that motivation toward a single health-related activity may leverage more than 1 pillar with a potentially reinforcing effect. Walking groups are a good example, as the experience boosts positive emotions from connecting with others (P), the feeling of flow of doing the physical activity (E), building relationships (R), developing meaning by keeping others accountable (M), and a sense of accomplishment when finished (A).

RESEARCH NEEDS

More research is needed on how intrinsic motivators vary and evolve across the lifespan, and which events and transition points lead to these motivators being more are malleable, for example, after an illness event. When will individuals respond to certain facilitators and when are individuals more sensitive to barriers, requiring additional assistance and support? Each individual's level of optimism, hope, personal strengths, risk-taking, and grit intersects with their stress levels, coping skills, emotional states, and personalities in the context of community and environmental influencers to determine health behaviors. How these factors evolve over the life course and how they interact need further investigation. Practical, evidence-based solutions for older adults along the spectrum of cognitive function are also required.

DISCUSSION

The essential steps in behavior change, such as autonomous goal setting, monitoring progress, and building self-efficacy are applicable across the lifespan, including aging individuals. Also, the counseling techniques, including MI, CBT, appreciative inquiry, and positive psychology (PP) can be effective methods of behavior change in older adults. In fact, due to generally better self-regulation, greater intrinsic motivators for psychological and physical well-being, these methods might be more effective in older adults than in their younger counterparts.

Building meaning into action steps and changes, as well as social support, are at the heart of change in all age groups, and are especially important in older adults. In addition, compensation for cognitive decline needs to be offered, such as helping to ensure adequate sleep and use of memory aids (handwritten notes, or built in reminders on phone devices, if used).

To effectively support health behavior change in older adults, methods to address the full spectrum of cognitive functioning needs to be considered and addressed, including working with caregivers. Further research is needed to refine coaching approaches across all age groups. Fortunately, existing health behavior change tools and approaches can be effective in adults experiencing a normal aging process to support well-being and achieve their "best self," even late in life.

DISCLOSURE

The author has nothing to disclose.

REFERENCES

1. Martin LR, Haskard-Zolnierek KB, DiMatteo MR. Health behavior change and treatment adherence: evidence-based guidelines for improving healthcare. Oxford (England): Oxford University Press; 2010. p. 157–75, 24–68, 51–68.
2. Lucas RE, Donnellan MB. Age differences in personality: evidence from a nationally representative Australian sample. Dev Psychol 2009;45(5):1353–63.
3. McCrae RR, Costa PT, Pedroso de Lima MP, et al. Age differences in personality across the adult life span: parallels in five cultures. Developmental Psychology 1999;35(2):466–77.
4. Glasgow RE, Nutting P. Diabetes. In: Hass LJ, editor. Handbook of primary care psychology. New York: Oxford University press; 2004. p. 299–311.
5. Egger G, Binns A, Rossner S. Lifestyle medicine: managing diseases of lifestyle in the 21st century. 2nd edition. Sydney (Australia): McGraw-Hill; 2011. p. 32–57.

6. Seligman MEP. Flourish: a visionary new understanding of happiness and well-being. New York City: Simon and Schuster; 2011.

7. Carstensen LL. The influence of a sense of time on human development. Science 2006;312(5782):1913–5.

8. Stone AA, Schwartz JE, Broderick JE, et al. A snapshot of the age distribution of psychological well-being in the United States. Proc Natl Acad Sci U S A 2010; 107(22):9985–90.

9. Carstensen LL, Turan B, Scheibe S, et al. Emotional experience improves with age: evidence based on over 10 years of experience sampling. Psychol Aging 2011;26(1):21–33.

10. Carstensen LL, Isaacowitz DM, Charles ST. Taking time seriously. A theory of socioemotional selectivity. *Am* Psychol 1999;54(3):165–81.

11. Heckausen J, Wrosch C, Schulz R. A motivational theory of life-span development. Psychol Rev 2010;117(1):32–60.

12. Charles ST. Strength and vulnerability integration: a model of emotional well-being across adulthood. Psychol Bull 2010;136(6):1068–91.

13. National Research Council (US) Committee on Aging in Social Psychology, Personality and Adult Developmental Psychology. In: Carstensen LL, Hartel CR, editors. When I'm 64. Washington, DC: National Academies Press (US); 2006.

14. Cabeza R, Daselaar SM, Dolcos F, et al. Task-dependent and task-specific age effects on brain activity during working memory, visual attention and episodic retrieval. Cereb Cortex 2004;14:364–75.

15. Logan JM, Sanders AL, Snyder AZ, et al. Under-recruitment and non-selective recruitment: dissociable neural mechanisms associated with aging. Neuron 2002;33:827–40.

16. Nielsen L, Reiss D. Motivation and aging: toward the next generation of behavioral interventions. Washington, DC: Division of Behavioral and Social Research, National Institute on Aging, NIA-BBCSS Expert Meeting Presentation; 2012.

17. Centers for Disease Control and Prevention, US Department of Health and Human Services. Writing SMART objectives. CDC Guide; Evaluation Briefs. No. 3b, 2018.

18. Grant AM, Cavanagh MJ. Evidence-based coaching: flourishing or languishing? Aust Psychol 2007;42(4):239–54.

19. Artinian NT, Fletcher GF, Mozaffarian D, et al. Interventions to promote physical activity and dietary lifestyle changes for cardiovascular risk factor reduction in adults: a scientific statement from the American Heart Association. Circulation 2010;122(4):406–41.

20. Elder JP, Ayala GX, Harris S. Theories and intervention approaches to health-behavior change in primary care. Am J Prev Med 1999;17(4):275–84.

21. National Cancer Institute. Theory at a glance: a guide for health promotion practice. Bethesda (MD): National Institutes of Health, National Cancer Institute; 1995. NIH Publication No. 95-3896.

22. Orleans CT. Treating nicotine dependence in medical settings. In: Orleans CT, Slade J, editors. Nicotine addiction: principles and management. New York: Oxford University Press; 1993. p. 148–50.

23. Lianov L. My happy avatar: use your mobile device and personality to transform your health. Sacramento (CA): HealthType; 2013.

24. Hill B, Richardson B, Skouteris H. Do we know how to design effective health coaching interventions: a systematic review of the state of the literature. Am J Health Promot 2015;29(5):e158–68.

25. Terry PE, Seaverson EL, Grossmeier J, et al. Effectiveness of a worksite telephone-based weight management program. Am J Health Promot 2011; 25(3):186–9.

26. Alley S, Jennings C, Plotnikoff RC, et al. Web-based video-coaching to assist an automated computer-tailored physical activity intervention for inactive adults: a randomized controlled trial. J Med Internet Res 2016;18(8):e223.

27. Dennison L, Morrison L, Lloyd S, et al. Does brief telephone support improve engagement with a web-based weight management intervention? Randomized controlled trial. J Med Internet Res 2014;16(3):e95.

28. Olsen JM, Nesbitt BJ. Health coaching to improve healthy lifestyle behaviors: an integrative review. Am J Health Promot 2010;25(1):e1–12.

29. Allman-Farinelli M, Partridge SR, McGeechan K, et al. A mobile health lifestyle program for prevention of weight gain in young adults (TXT2BFiT): nine-month outcomes of a randomized controlled trial. JMIR Mhealth Uhealth 2016;4(2):e78.

30. Bennett GG, Herring SJ, Puleo E, et al. Web-based weight loss in primary care: a randomized controlled trial. *Obesity* (Silver Spring) 2010;18(2):308–13.

31. Kivelä K, Elo S, Kyngäs H, et al. The effects of health coaching on adult patients with chronic diseases: a systematic review. Patient Educ Couns 2014;97(2): 147–57.

32. Mao AY, Chen C, Magana C, et al. A mobile phone-based health coaching intervention for weight loss and blood pressure reduction in a national payer population: a retrospective study. JMIR Mhealth Uhealth 2017;5(6):e80.

33. Wayne N, Perez DF, Kaplan DM, et al. Health coaching reduces HbA1c in type 2 diabetic patients from a lower-socioeconomic status community: a randomized controlled trial. J Med Internet Res 2015;17(10):e224.

34. Newnham-Kanas C, Gorczynski P, Morrow D, et al. Annotated bibliography of life coaching and health research. Int J Evid Based Coach Mentor 2009;7(1):39–103.

35. Quinn CC, Shardell MD, Terrin ML, et al. Cluster-randomized trial of a mobile phone personalized behavioral intervention for blood glucose control. Diabetes Care 2011;34(9):1934–42.

36. Wolever RQ, Dreusicke M, Fikkan J, et al. Integrative health coaching for patients with type 2 diabetes: a randomized clinical trial. Diabetes Educ 2010;36(4): 629–39.

37. Hutchison AJ, Breckon JD. A review of telephone coaching services for people with long-term conditions. J Telemed Telecare 2011;17(8):451–8.

38. Lianov L. Roots of positive change: optimizing health car with positive psychology. Chesterfield (MO): American College of Lifestyle Medicine; 2019.

39. Spahn JM, Reeves RS, Keim KS, et al. State of the evidence regarding behavior change theories and strategies in nutrition counseling to facilitate health and food behavior change. J Am Diet Assoc 2010;110(6):879–91.

40. Prochaska JO, DiClemente CC. Stages and processes of self-change of smoking: toward an integrative model of change. J Consult Clin Psychol 1983;51(3): 390–5.

41. Quindry JC, Yount D, O'Bryant H, et al. Exercise engagement is differentially motivated by age-dependent factors. Am J Health Behav 2011;35(3):334–45.

42. Gholami M, Herman C, Ainsworth MC, et al. Applying Psychological Theories to Promote Healthy Lifestyles. In: Rippe JM, editor. *Lifestyle Medicine. 3rd edition.* p. 197-217.

43. Abrams DB, Emons KM, Linnan LA. Health behavior and health education: the past, present, and future. In: Glanz K, Lewis F, Rimer B, editors. Health behavior

and health education: theory, research, and practice. 2nd ediiton. San Francisco (CA): Jossey; 1999. p. 453–7.

44. Heaney CA, Israil BA. Social networks and social support. In: Glanz K, Lewis F, Rimer B, editors. Health behavior and health education: theory, research, and practice. San Francisco (CA): Jossey-Bass; 1999. p. 179–205.

45. Abrams DB, Orleans CT, Niavra RS, et al. Integrating individual and public health perspectives for treatment of tobacco dependency in managed care: a combined stepped-care and matching model. Ann Behav Med 1996;10(4):20–304.

46. Harvard study of adult development. Available at: www.adultdevelopmentstudy. org. Accessed November 25, 2019.

47. Emmons KM, Rollnick S. Motivational interviewing in health care settings. Opportunities and limitations. Am J Prev Med 2001;20(1):68–74.

48. Simpson M, Buckman R, Stewart M, et al. Doctor-patient communication: the Toronto consensus statement. Br Med J 1991;303(6814):1385–7.

49. Anderson GO. Technology use and attitudes among mid-life and older Americans. Washington, DC: American Association of Retired Persons; 2017.

50. Mander BA, Rao V, Lu B, et al. Prefrontal atrophy, disrupted NREM slow waved, and impaired hippocampal-dependent memory in aging. Nat Neurosci 2013; 16(3):357–64.

51. Hojat M, Mangione S, Nasca TJ, et al. Empathy scores in medical school and ratings of empathetic behavior in residency training 3 years later. The Journal of Social Psychology 2010;145(6):663–72.

52. Chaitoff A, Rothberg MB, Martinez KA. Physician empathy and diabetes outcomes. J Gen Intern Med. 2019;34(10):1967.

53. Miller WR, Rollnick S. Motivational interviewing: preparing people for change. 2nd ediiton. New York: Guilford Press; 2002.

54. Fifield P, Susuki J, Minski S, et al. Motivational interviewing and lifestyle change. In: Rippe JM, editor. Lifestyle medicine. 3rd edition. Boca Raton (FL): CRC Press, Taylor & Francis Group; 2019. p. 207–17.

55. Rollnick S, Mason P, Butler C. Health behavior change: a guide for practitioners. Edinburgh (UK): Churchill Livingstone; 2003. p. 73–104.

56. Lundhahl B, Burke BL. The effectiveness and applicability of motivational interviewing: a practice-friendly review of four meta-analysis. J Clin Psychol 2009; 65(11):1232–45.

57. Acosta AS, Douthwaite B. Appreciative Inquiry: An approach for learning and change based on our best practices. ILAC Brief 6. p. 1-4

58. Frates B, Bonnet JP, Joseph R, et al. Lifestyle medicine handbook: an introduction to the power of healthy habits. Monterey (CA): Healthy Learning; 2019. p. 97–9.

59. Guide to Community Preventive Services. Behavioral and social approaches to increase physical activity: individually-adapted health behavior change programs. Available at: www.thecommunityguide.org/pa/behavioral-social/ individuallyadapted.html. Accessed July 17, 2020.

60. Thompson RS. What have HMOs learned about clinical preventive services? An examination of the experience at Group Health Cooperative of Puget Soud. Milbank Q 1996;74(4):469–509.

61. Miller WR, Rollnick S. Motivational interviewing: preparing people to change addictive behavior. New York: Guildford Press; 1991.

62. Ad Hoc Committee on Health Literacy for the Council on Scientific Affairs. Health literacy: Report of the Council on Scientific Affairs. JAMA 1999;281(6):552–7.

63. Lerman CE, Brody DS, Caputo GC, et al. Patients' perceived involvement in care scale: relationship to attitudes about illness and medical care. J Gen Intern Med 1990;5(1):29–33.
64. Miller WR. Enhancing motivation for change. In: Miller WR, Heather N, DS, editors. Treating addictive behaviors. 2nd edition. New York: Premium Press; 1998. p. 121–32.
65. Donovan JL, Blake DR. Patient non-compliance: deviance or reasoned decision-making? Soc Sci Med 1992;34(5):507–13.
66. Bandura A. Social foundations of thought and action: a social cognitive theory. Englewood Cliffs (NJ): Prentice Hall; 1986.
67. Orleans CT. Promoting the maintenance of health behavior change: Recommendations for the next generation of research and practice. Health Psychol 2000; 19(supple 1):76–83.
68. Donovan DL. Continuing care: promoting the maintenance of change. In: Miller WR, Heather N, DS, editors. Treating addictive behaviors. New York: Plenum Press; 1998. p. 317–37.
69. Biswas-Diener R. Practicing positive psychology coaching: assessment, activities and strategies for success. Hoboken (NJ): John Wiley & Sons; 2012.
70. Kaufman C. Positive psychology: the science at the heart of coaching. In: Stober D, Grant A, editors. Evidence-based coaching: putting best practices to work for your clients. Hoboken (NJ): John Wiley & Sons; 2006. p. 219–53.
71. McQuaid M, Niemiec R, Doman F. A character strengths-based approach to positive psychology. Positive Psychology Coaching for Health and Wellbeing. In: Green S, Palmer S, editors. Rutledge, Positive Psychology Coaching in Practice. Oxford (United Kingdom): 2019.
72. Boyatzis RE, Akrivou K. The ideal self as the driver of intentional change. J Manage Development 2006;25(7):624–42.
73. Park N, Peterson C. Character strengths: research and practice. J Coll Character 2009;10(4).
74. Values in action survey. Available at: http://www.viacharacter.org. Accessed July 17, 2020.
75. Fredrickson BL. Positive emotions broaden and build. Advances in experimental social psychology. Acad Press 2013;47:1–53.
76. Van Cappellen P, Rice EL, Catalino LI, et al. Positive affective processes underlie positive health behavior change. Psychol Health 2018;33(1):77–97.
77. Palmer S, Green S. PERMA-powered coaching:Building foundations for a flourishing life. Positive Psychology Coaching in Practice 2018;125–42.

UNITED STATES POSTAL SERVICE ® Statement of Ownership, Management, and Circulation (All Periodicals Publications Except Requester Publications)

1. Publication Title	2. Publication Number	3. Filing Date
CLINICS IN GERIATRIC MEDICINE	000 – 704	9/18/2020

4. Issue Frequency	5. Number of Issues Published Annually	6. Annual Subscription Price
FEB, MAY, AUG, NOV	4	$289.00

7. Complete Mailing Address of Known Office of Publication (Not printer) (Street, city, county, state, and ZIP+4®)

ELSEVIER INC.
230 Park Avenue, Suite 800
New York, NY 10169

Contact Person
Malathi Samayan

Telephone (Include area code)
91-44-4299-4507

8. Complete Mailing Address of Headquarters or General Business Office of Publisher (Not printer)

ELSEVIER INC.
230 Park Avenue, Suite 800
New York, NY 10169

9. Full Names and Complete Mailing Addresses of Publisher, Editor, and Managing Editor (Do not leave blank)

Publisher (Name and complete mailing address)

DOLORES MELONI, ELSEVIER INC.
1600 JOHN F KENNEDY BLVD. SUITE 1800
PHILADELPHIA, PA 19103-2899

Editor (Name and complete mailing address)

KATERINA HEIDHAUSEN, ELSEVIER INC.
1600 JOHN F KENNEDY BLVD. SUITE 1800
PHILADELPHIA, PA 19103-2899

Managing Editor (Name and complete mailing address)

PATRICK MANLEY, ELSEVIER INC.
1600 JOHN F KENNEDY BLVD. SUITE 1800
PHILADELPHIA, PA 19103-2899

10. Owner (Do not leave blank. If the publication is owned by a corporation, give the name and address of the corporation immediately followed by the names and addresses of all stockholders owning or holding 1 percent or more of the total amount of stock. If not owned by a corporation, give the names and addresses of the individual owners. If owned by a partnership or other unincorporated firm, give its name and address as well as those of each individual owner. If the publication is published by a nonprofit organization, give its name and address.)

Full Name	Complete Mailing Address
WHOLLY OWNED SUBSIDIARY OF REED/ELSEVIER, US HOLDINGS	1600 JOHN F KENNEDY BLVD. SUITE 1800 PHILADELPHIA, PA 19103-2899

11. Known Bondholders, Mortgagees, and Other Security Holders Owning or Holding 1 Percent or More of Total Amount of Bonds, Mortgages, or Other Securities. If none, check box ▸ ☐ None

Full Name	Complete Mailing Address
N/A	

12. Tax Status (For completion by nonprofit organizations authorized to mail at nonprofit rates) (Check one)
The purpose, function, and nonprofit status of this organization and the exempt status for federal income tax purposes:
☒ Has Not Changed During Preceding 12 Months
☐ Has Changed During Preceding 12 Months (Publisher must submit explanation of change with this statement)

PS Form 3526, July 2014 [Page 1 of 4 (see instructions page 4)]   PSN 7530-01-000-9931   PRIVACY NOTICE: See our privacy policy on www.usps.com

13. Publication Title	14. Issue Date for Circulation Data Below
CLINICS IN GERIATRIC MEDICINE	MAY 2020

15. Extent and Nature of Circulation		Average No. Copies Each Issue During Preceding 12 Months	No. Copies of Single Issue Published Nearest to Filing Date
a. Total Number of Copies (Net press run)		143	122
b. Paid Circulation (By Mail and Outside the Mail)	(1) Mailed Outside-County Paid Subscriptions Stated on PS Form 3541 (include paid distribution above nominal rate, advertiser's proof copies, and exchange copies)	69	65
	(2) Mailed In-County Paid Subscriptions Stated on PS Form 3541 (Include paid distribution above nominal rate, advertiser's proof copies, and exchange copies)	0	0
	(3) Paid Distribution Outside the Mails Including Sales Through Dealers and Carriers, Street Vendors, Counter Sales, and Other Paid Distribution Outside USPS®	31	29
	(4) Paid Distribution by Other Classes of Mail Through the USPS (e.g. First-Class Mail®)	0	0
c. Total Paid Distribution (Sum of 15b (1), (2), (3), and (4)) ▸		100	94
d. Free or Nominal Rate Distribution (By Mail and Outside the Mail)	(1) Free or Nominal Rate Outside-County Copies included on PS Form 3541	29	11
	(2) Free or Nominal Rate In-County Copies Included on PS Form 3541	0	0
	(3) Free or Nominal Rate Copies Mailed at Other Classes Through the USPS (e.g. First-Class Mail)	0	0
	(4) Free or Nominal Rate Distribution Outside the Mail (Carriers or other means)	29	11
e. Total Free or Nominal Rate Distribution (Sum of 15d (1), (2), (3) and (4)) ▸		29	11
f. Total Distribution (Sum of 15c and 15e) ▸		129	105
g. Copies not Distributed (See Instructions to Publishers #4 (page #3)) ▸		14	17
h. Total (Sum of 15f and g) ▸		143	122
i. Percent Paid (15c divided by 15f times 100) ▸		77.51%	89.52%

* If you are claiming electronic copies, go to line 16 on page 3. If you are not claiming electronic copies, skip to line 17 on page 3.

16. Electronic Copy Circulation		Average No. Copies Each Issue During Preceding 12 Months	No. Copies of Single Issue Published Nearest to Filing Date
a. Paid Electronic Copies ▸			
b. Total Paid Print Copies (Line 15c) + Paid Electronic Copies (Line 16a) ▸			
c. Total Print Distribution (Line 15f) + Paid Electronic Copies (Line 16a) ▸			
d. Percent Paid (Both Print & Electronic Copies) (16b divided by 16c × 100) ▸			

☒ I certify that 50% of all my distributed copies (electronic and print) are paid above a nominal price.

17. Publication of Statement of Ownership

☒ If the publication is a general publication, publication of this statement is required. Will be printed
in the NOVEMBER 2020 issue of this publication.   ☐ Publication not required.

18. Signature and Title of Editor, Publisher, Business Manager, or Owner

Malathi Samayan - Distribution Controller   *Malathi Samayan*

Date 9/18/2020

I certify that all information furnished on this form is true and complete. I understand that anyone who furnishes false or misleading information on this form or who omits material or information requested on the form may be subject to criminal sanctions (including fines and imprisonment) and/or civil sanctions (including civil penalties).

PS Form 3526, July 2014 (Page 3 of 4)   PRIVACY NOTICE: See our privacy policy on www.usps.com

Printed and bound by CPI Group (UK) Ltd, Croydon, CR0 4YY

03/10/2024

01040404-0017